WISDOM IN PSYCHIATRY

UNDERSTANDING BEGINS HEALING

RAVINDER NATH BHALLA MD

This book is a work of creative nonfiction. Clinical material is drawn from real encounters but presented in composite, anonymized, or otherwise altered form to protect confidentiality. Any resemblance to actual individuals is coincidental and unintentional.

For permissions or inquiries, contact: drravibhalla@gmail.com

Printed in the United States.

ISBN: 978-1-971562-01-8 paperback

ISBN: 978-1-971562-02-5 hard

ISBN: 978-1-971562-00-1 ebook

~

To my patients—
who have revealed courage in its quietest forms
and taught me more about the mind
than any training ever could.
And to those who still suffer in silence:
may you find language, companionship,
and the wisdom that heals.

~

ACKNOWLEDGMENTS

A book like this is not written alone. It accumulates — over years, across rooms, through encounters that leave their mark long after the conversation ends.

I am grateful, first, to my patients. You trusted me with what was unfinished, uncertain, and often unspeakable. You taught me that healing rarely follows a straight line, and that being understood sometimes matters more than being cured. Whatever insight lives in these pages began with you.

To my colleagues and mentors — those who challenged my assumptions, sharpened my thinking, and reminded me that humility is not weakness but necessity — thank you. Psychiatry is refined in dialogue, and I have been fortunate in my teachers.

To my family — for your patience, your faith, and your steady presence through the long hours — I owe more than these words can hold.

And to the years themselves: the slow accumulation of experience that becomes, if one is attentive and lucky, something resembling wisdom. I did not always understand what I was learning. I am still learning now.

∾

CONTENTS

PART II

PART III

PART IV

PART V

PREFACE

What I Learned Over the Years

This book was not planned. It accumulated slowly—through thousands of clinical hours, through the quiet of my office after the last patient left, through questions that stayed with me long after a diagnosis had been given and a note closed.

Early in my career, the central challenge of psychiatry was identifying the correct condition. If the diagnoses were accurate, I thought, the treatment would follow and improvement would unfold. Our tools—interviews, manuals, medications, psychotherapies—seemed sufficient.

I no longer believe this.

Nothing dramatically changed my mind. There was no single catastrophic case. Instead, something more subtle happened: a slow accumulation of unease. A child who returned months later, largely unchanged, despite my confidence in the treatment plan. A teenager whose symptoms only made sense to me years after she had dropped out of therapy. A parent who quietly admitted she had never really understood her son's diagnosis but was too ashamed to say so earlier. A young adult who nodded politely in every session yet seemed to live in a private world I never quite reached.

These were not failures of intelligence, effort, or training. They were failures of understanding. Failures of seeing.

The Missing Element

There is a kind of wisdom one acquires only with time—when patterns of human suffering begin to emerge more clearly, when the limits of technical expertise become undeniable, and when one has lived long enough to witness the long arc of patients' lives beyond the initial consultation.

This is the wisdom I wish I had earlier: the wisdom to listen more slowly, to question my first impressions, to be wary of diagnostic confidence, to recognize the emotional weight patients pack into simple words, to see when my own biases were shaping the narrative, to notice when a patient agreed only to preserve dignity, to sense when silence contained more truth than speech, to understand that "noncompliance" was often a form of pain, and to recognize that stigma, culture, and family expectations were shaping treatment as much as biology.

Wisdom in psychiatry is not ornamental. It is essential. And yet no residency program teaches it. No manual contains it. No checklist can capture it. In truth, wisdom is acquired the way many patients heal: slowly, unevenly, with humility, and sometimes with regret.

Why I Am Writing This Book Now

I am writing because I have arrived at a vantage point from which the whole arc of my career is visible—its successes, its blind spots, its mistakes, and its unanswered questions.

I am writing because I have come to see that diagnosis is not merely a scientific act. It is also human, one— shaped by communication, culture, fear, and interpretation.

I am writing because I have watched too many patients suffer unnecessarily from miscommunication, misunderstanding, and misalignment between diagnosis and treatment.

I am writing because clinicians rarely speak openly about uncertainty, and patients rarely hear that uncertainty can be part of wise care, not evidence of incompetence.

I am writing because psychiatry's future will almost certainly include more powerful technologies—and I fear that without deeper human insight; those tools will sharpen our errors as easily as our truths.

And I am writing because I have seen what becomes possible when a clinician approaches a patient with openness, courage, and the humility to admit that words are poor representations of thoughts, and even poorer representations of feelings.

A Word on Nietzsche

Readers will notice the presence of Friedrich Nietzsche throughout this book.

He is not here as a distant philosopher to be worshipped. He is here because his insights illuminate something at the center of psychiatric work: we are shaped—and often trapped—by the interpretations we inherit and the language we use to describe ourselves.

Nietzsche understood that human beings are, above all, makers of meaning. In psychiatry, we must add- human beings are also *defenders* of meaning. They protect fragile identities with silence, euphemism, denial, or borrowed explanations.

Nietzsche reminds us that the difficulty of seeing oneself clearly is a universal struggle, not a clinical defect. His presence in these pages will be modest but purposeful: a guide in thinking about self-deception, the limits of language, the struggle for self-knowledge, the courage required for transformation, and the weight of societal expectation. In this sense, he stands beside us—not above us—as we try to understand how people come to misname their own suffering and how we, as clinicians, sometimes help them do it.

What This Book Is—and Is Not

This is not a textbook. It is not a diagnostic manual. It is not a wholesale critique of psychiatry, though it contains critique. It is not a memoir, though it is shaped by my experience.

This book is an exploration—of the space between what patients express and what clinicians understand, of the distortions that enter every clinical encounter, and of the kind of wisdom required to navigate them.

It is meant for clinicians who sense that something essential is missing from their training. For patients who want to understand what happens on the other side of the desk. For parents, partners, teachers, and caregivers who are trying to comprehend the inner lives of those they love. And for any thoughtful reader seeking a deeper understanding of mental suffering.

Over the decades, I have learned that truly seeing a patient requires more than knowledge. It requires a way of being- slower, more curious, less defensive, more willing to be changed by what one learns.

This book is an invitation into that way.

A Final Note of Gratitude

To the patients I have treated over the years: you are the true authors of this book. From each of you, I have learned something I could not have learned otherwise. Your courage, your silences, your metaphors, your refusals—all of it has shaped my understanding of the human mind.

This book is dedicated to the possibility that we might understand one another a little more clearly—and suffer a little less because of it.

∾

INTRODUCTION

INTRODUCTION — Words and the Space Around Them

From the very beginning of my career— and in nearly every clinical room I've stepped into since—patients have arrived already holding two familiar words: *depression* and *anxiety*. Words handed to them by previous clinicians, by the internet, by relatives, by the culture itself. Words they learned to use because they were recognizable and safe, not because they captured the truth.

A patient would sit down, fold their hands neatly, and say, "I have depression... and anxiety." And somewhere in their chart, a well-meaning clinician had precisely written- Major Depression with Anxiety. A tidy diagnosis was born from tidy language.

But these two words soon revealed themselves as some of the most misleading in our field.

One patient used *anxiety* to describe the soft flutter that came before a presentation. Another used the same word to describe a private free-fall—heart racing, chest tightening, the terrifying conviction that he was disappearing from his own life.

Same word. Different universe.

It was then I began asking every patient—gently, consistently: "Tell me how you suffer without using the words depression or anxiety. Not with me, and also not with any other doctor. Tell me how it feels in your body, in your hours, in your days."

At first, they would hesitate, caught off guard, unsure how to speak without the protective mask of those familiar labels. But gradually, they would reach for language that was raw, personal, revealing.

A woman once said, "It feels like my bones are tired." A man whispered, "It feels like the ground beneath me is humming too loudly." Another said, "It feels like my thoughts are trying to outrun me." Someone else described, "It feels like someone drained all the color from my life."

These were not diagnoses. They were experiences— unfiltered and unclipped by medical vocabulary. They carried a truth no checklist could detect.

This practice became the least I could do to prevent the quiet slide into miscommunication and misdiagnosis. Because once a patient defaults to "depression" or "anxiety," the clinician hears a category, not a person. And the person disappears behind the shorthand.

There is always a distance between what a person feels and what they can bring themselves to say. Not an empty distance, but a terrain— uneven, shaped by childhood, culture, shame, hope, and all the unspoken rules that govern emotional life.

Words cross this terrain imperfectly. They do not carry the feeling; they only gesture toward it.

By the time a patient speaks, their experience has already passed through filters: family expectations, cultural scripts, private fears, the instinct to appear controlled, the dread of being misunderstood. What reaches the clinician is the part that survived translation.

And yet, we diagnose based on these words.

Over time, I learned to listen not only to what patients said but to the places where language failed them: the pauses, the contradictions, the protective laughter, the metaphors chosen in desperation. Wisdom in psychiatry is the ability to listen to words *and* the space around them— the struggle, silence, the self-protection.

Training teaches technique. Experience teaches humility. Wisdom teaches the limits of language.

Two people can sit in the same room, speak the same language, and mean entirely different things. Diagnosis depends on words. Understanding depends on interpreting the human being beneath those words.

Our diagnostic systems were built for clarity, but the human mind refuses to be made neat. Symptoms overlap. Trauma hides beneath socially acceptable language. Culture shapes what can be said and what must remain unspoken. People bury their most painful truths beneath words that feel safe.

Without wisdom, psychiatry becomes an enterprise of partial truths—accurate enough to justify treatment, too thin to illuminate its origins.

This book explores the unreliable space around words: the gap between what is felt and what is named, what is named and what is understood.

It is not a rejection of science. It is an appeal for depth.

For a psychiatry that treats diagnosis as interpretation, not verdict. For a discipline that listens for the private meanings beneath public language.

Healing begins not when a symptom is labeled, but when a person finally feels understood—when their inner world, long mistranslated, finds a language that fits.

And so, we begin here, in the trembling space around words, where meaning slips, reforms, and reveals itself—quietly, like breath returning after a long hold.

∼

VOLUME ONE

WISDOM IN INTERVIEWING

PART I

The Burden of Misunderstanding

Before we can see clearly, we must understand why we so often see wrongly.

Psychiatric encounters begin in uncertainty. Words fail. Bias intrudes. Conclusions arrive too quickly.

Part I examines the forces that distort clinical perception — and reveals why wisdom must precede technique.

1

WHY PSYCHIATRY NEEDS WISDOM

*"We are always in flight from the truth that would demand our
transformation."*
— Friedrich Nietzsche

Psychiatry presents itself as a discipline of answers—
diagnoses drawn from criteria, treatments organized into
protocols, outcomes measured through metrics. Yet
beneath that appearance of precision lies a more fragile truth: every
clinical encounter begins in uncertainty.

Two human beings sit across from each other, each shaped by
their histories, their biases, their longings, and their fears. One seeks
relief; the other seeks understanding. What unfolds between them is
not algorithmic. It is interpretive. It is emotional. It is human.

Wisdom is not decoration in this work—it is its foundation.
Without it, we risk hearing words but missing meaning, following
protocols while overlooking contradictions, diagnosing accurately yet
relieving little suffering. Wisdom slows the clinician's mind, softens

certainty, and amplifies perception. It allows us to see the person behind the presentation.

EARLY IN MY CAREER, I believed knowledge alone would suffice. I memorized criteria, differentiated disorders, and mastered checklists. But knowledge is narrow. It notices what fits the model and discards what falls outside it. Human beings rarely fall neatly inside anything. They overflow, compress, disguise, and translate their experiences— often unconsciously—into forms they believe will be acceptable.

One of my earliest lessons came from a woman who appeared to have a straightforward depressive episode—flat affect, insomnia, hopelessness. Everything fits. But her sadness felt practiced, as if she were offering the version of herself, she assumed I needed to see. It wasn't until later, after trust had grown, that she revealed flashes of agitation: racing thoughts, surges of energy, an undercurrent of rest-lessness. She was not simply depressed; she was edging toward a mixed manic state. Had I treated her initial story as the complete one, I would have caused harm.

That moment marked my first true encounter with clinical humil-ity. Patients rarely begin with the truth that hurts the most; they begin with the truth they believe is speakable. Wisdom is the clinician's capacity to recognize this difference—not through suspicion, but through openness.

WISDOM ASKS us to hold diagnosis lightly at first. To listen for the emotional, cultural, and developmental layers beneath the patient's words. To sense when language has not yet caught up with experi-ence. To remain curious when everything in us urges quick certainty.

Nietzsche wrote, "We remain unknown to ourselves." In psychiatry, this is not merely a philosophical observation— it is a daily reality. Patients are often strangers to their own interior world, narrating themselves through borrowed language, family stories, or cultural scripts. Clinicians, too, are vulnerable to their own blind spots: confirmation bias, premature closure, the illusion of mastery.

Wisdom, then, is a counterbalance. It widens perception, slows interpretation, and interrupts the clinician's urge to finalize an understanding before it has fully formed.

This is why the Nietzsche epigraph opens this chapter. People instinctively protect themselves from truths that require emotional change. The patient flees from painful self-knowledge; the clinician flees from the discomfort of not knowing. Wisdom is needed precisely because the mind hides exactly what most needs to be seen —in both parties.

SYMPTOMS LIE—NOT intentionally, but structurally. They are surface expressions of deeper processes: trauma, identity conflict, shame, grief, unspoken need, cultural restraint. Treating symptoms alone is like treating the reflection in a mirror rather than the person standing before it.

Years later, I met a middle-aged man referred for classic panic attacks: racing heart, trembling, fear of losing control. His description was textbook. But something in his voice—its resignation, its careful neutrality—felt like a veil. His panic was real, but it was also a shield. Beneath it lay decades of unresolved grief: the silent sorrow of a father who had died without ever acknowledging him. His body expressed what his voice had been forbidden to speak.

Wisdom asked the question the diagnosis could not: What is the panic protecting?

Only then could healing begin.

. . .

WISDOM TEACHES us to attend to what is absent as much as to what is present: the missing emotion, the too-neat narrative, the smile that avoids the eyes. It teaches us to notice when shame shapes a patient's account, when culture restricts disclosure, when trauma distorts memory, when hope hides inside fear.

Over the years, I reviewed the work of other practitioners— good, well-intentioned clinicians—and saw a common struggle: difficulty course-correcting. Once a diagnosis had been named, it clung stubbornly, even when the patient's improvement stalled or worsened. Confirmation bias and the comfort of familiarity often kept both patient and clinician locked in outdated interpretations.

Wisdom resists such rigidity. It asks the clinician to return again and again to the essential questions: Is my understanding still accurate? Is this treatment still, right? What am I missing? Wisdom values seeing over assuming, evolving over clinging, healing over defending one's own correctness.

In this way, wisdom becomes less a trait than a discipline—a way of perceiving, a stance toward uncertainty, a commitment to understanding the unseen forces shaping a patient's suffering.

Only through such widened seeing can psychiatry move toward its deepest aim: not simply to diagnose, but to truly understand.

~

2

THE POVERTY OF WORDS

"Truths are illusions of which one has forgotten that they are illusions."
— Friedrich Nietzsche

Words are small containers for large experiences.

People arrive in the clinic carrying lifetimes—grief sedimented into the body, fears inherited across generations, identities shaped by culture, temperament, and circumstance. Yet when asked to speak, they must compress all of this into a handful of sentences. What they offer is not the truth of their suffering, but the version of it that language can hold.

In psychiatry, we depend on words to guide diagnosis, but words deceive us by omission. They reveal only the layers a patient is able—or willing—to articulate. The rest remains submerged: memories without language, emotions without narrative, sensations without meaning. Even the most honest patient speaks in approximation.

A person may describe sadness when they mean despair, anxiety when they mean dread, trauma when they mean violation. Even the most precise vocabulary cannot fully express what the body knows. The language of suffering is always partial because suffering itself resists containment.

I ONCE SAW a young woman in her early twenties who told me, "I don't feel like myself."

It was a vague phrase; one used so casually in ordinary life that it barely seemed diagnostic. But the heaviness behind it— her flattened gaze, her taut stillness—suggested something deeper. When I asked what she meant, she repeated the same words, quieter this time, as though afraid of hearing herself speak.

Only months later did she reveal what she could not articulate then: that "not myself" meant a dissociation rooted in childhood experiences she had never named, not even privately. Her vocabulary had been too fragile to hold her truth.

This is the poverty of words: the gap between what is lived and what is said.

LANGUAGE IS SHAPED BY CULTURE, by family norms, by what has been permissible or safe to express.

A child raised in a home where emotions were punished grows into an adult who speaks in understatement. A person from a culture that somaticizes distress will speak through the body—headaches, dizziness, stomach pain—because emotional vocabulary is scarce or forbidden. Others overuse psychiatric terms, masking vulnerability behind clinical sophistication. The word *depression* becomes armor. The phrase *panic attack* becomes a way of saying something without revealing anything.

Clinicians, too, can misunderstand the limits of language. We ask for clarity as though clarity were always possible. We press for precision as though vocabulary were evenly distributed across lives. But people do not come to us being fluent in the language of their own suffering. Many have never been taught the words for what they feel. Others have been taught the wrong words—labels handed down by families or previous clinicians that obscured more than they revealed.

Wisdom requires a different kind of listening—one that attends not only to words but to the spaces around them. Hesitation before a response. The long inhale before admitting something painful. The moment the eyes drop when a patient contradicts themselves. These, too, are forms of communication—often truer than the sentences that follow.

A MAN once told me he felt "off."

When I asked him what he meant, he shrugged, embarrassed. For weeks he could not elaborate. Only through gentle, patient exploration did we uncover what lay beneath: a mix of depersonalization, chronic loneliness, and a quiet terror of becoming like his father, who had spiraled into psychosis.

"Off" was not avoidance. It was the only word he possessed to gesture toward a fear too large to name.

THE POVERTY of words is not a failure of the patient. It is a condition of being human.

Nietzsche captured this limitation in his reflections on language and metaphor, noting that words are merely worn-out symbols— poor representatives of thoughts, and thoughts themselves even poorer representatives of feeling. For him, language is not a mirror of reality but a set of approximations, distortions, and inherited conventions. In the clinic, we see this daily: what a patient feels arrives only as a distant echo of the original experience.

Nietzsche also warned that truths are illusions of which one has forgotten that they are illusions. Nowhere is this more evident than in psychiatric practice. A patient's words carry the authority of truth, yet beneath them lie older interpretations—shaped by childhood, culture, fear, and necessity—that have been repeated so long they feel factual. What we hear in the room is not the original experience but the story that has calcified around it.

This is why premature conclusions are so seductive. They protect both patient and clinician from the discomfort of uncertainty. They offer the relief of a name, a category, a path forward. But this haste creates an illusion of clarity, masking deeper truths that require patience to uncover. Psychiatric misdiagnosis is often the result of fleeing complexity, not a lack of intelligence or training.

The wise clinician resists this flight. Rather than listening to polished narratives, they listen around the rough edges of meaning—the contradictions, the silences, the places where language strains against experience. They listen to the story trying to take shape beneath the one being told.

∾

3

THE TWIN BIASES:
PATIENT AND CLINICIAN

"We see through the eyes of all our yesterdays."
— Friedrich Nietzsche

P atients rarely speak from a place of neutrality.

Their narratives are filtered through shame, fear of judgment, cultural norms, and the desire to present themselves in a way that preserves dignity. They edit, embellish, minimize, or reorganize their experiences depending on how safe they feel.

Some underreport symptoms because they fear being labeled. Some overreport because they fear being dismissed. Others offer clinically shaped language because they have learned that medical vocabulary earns seriousness. And some speak in metaphors because their distress has no direct linguistic form.

One patient with severe anxiety insisted that she was "fine." Her calm tone, steady posture, and careful grooming reinforced the illusion. Yet her hands trembled with the slightest movement. When I asked what "fine" meant to her, her eyes filled—not with tears, but with panic. She had grown up in a home where displaying distress was punished. Her words were obedient to her childhood, not to her present reality.

Patients do not lie—they protect. They protect themselves from the shame of being misunderstood, from the fear of being seen too clearly, from the threat of confirming what they most dread about themselves.

The Constraints of Expertise

Clinicians, for their part, enter sessions carrying their own limitations.

Training teaches us to think in patterns, to seek diagnostic landmarks, to match symptoms to criteria. This is necessary. But it also narrows perception. We hear familiar phrases and assume familiar disorders. We rely on the language we've mastered rather than the meaning emerging in real time. Our experience becomes a filter—we see what we've seen before, even when something entirely new is unfolding.

Overconfidence may be the most dangerous bias of all. The belief that we "know" what a patient means because their words resemble those of countless others blinds us to the individuality of suffering. Two patients may say they are depressed, yet their depressions may arise from entirely different emotional architectures.

Clinician bias also emerges from exhaustion, from the pressure to be efficient, from the subtle internal competition to make accurate diagnoses quickly. We rush too easily toward conclusions because uncertainty feels professionally uncomfortable.

Where the Biases Meet

Most misunderstandings in psychiatry arise in the space where these two biases collide. A patient filters their truth to protect themselves, while a clinician filters the patient's story through the lens of training and pattern recognition. What results is a partial understanding—accurate enough to begin treatment, but incomplete enough to miss the deeper forces shaping the patient's life.

A man once told me he was "angry all the time." I nearly followed the familiar path toward mood disorders, irritability, and stress-related dynamics. But something in his tone lacked true anger; it carried grief. When I asked him about the last time he felt this anger, he hesitated. His anger was not anger—it was sorrow that had calcified. Because he grew up in a family where sadness was forbidden, he had learned to rename it.

Had I followed my instinct, guided by training and experience alone, I would have treated anger. Wisdom, however, asked for pause.

This is why the Nietzsche epigraph opens this chapter. Patients speak through the emotional residue of their histories. Clinicians listen through the frameworks built by their training and their own past. Every misunderstanding in psychiatry begins when two histories collide—when what the patient needs to hide meets what the clinician expects to find.

WISDOM as the Corrective Lens

Wisdom does not eliminate bias; it reveals it.

It encourages clinicians to hold their interpretations loosely, to listen for the patient's emotional truth beneath their linguistic habits, to sense when shame or fear is shaping the story.

Nietzsche reminds us that there are no facts, only interpretations. In the clinical room, this is not a philosophical abstraction—it is a daily reality. A patient's narrative is an interpretation of their suffer-

ing; a clinician's understanding is an interpretation of that interpretation. Wisdom is the steadying force that keeps both from mistaking
first impressions for truth.

Bias becomes dangerous only when it goes unrecognized.
Wisdom—humble, patient, and emotionally attuned—keeps both
parties closer to the truth of their encounter.

When clinician and patient begin to recognize their biases,
understanding deepens. The conversation becomes less about symptoms and more about the human forces that give rise to them.

It is here, in this shared recognition, that healing begins.

THE COLLISION IN PRACTICE: Bipolar Depression Mistaken for
Unipolar

Consider how often bipolar depression is misdiagnosed as major
depression—a pattern so common it has become almost emblematic
of the hidden forces shaping clinical work.

The patient describes exhaustion, sadness, hopelessness, and the
clinician hears the familiar architecture of unipolar depression. Both
believe they are speaking the same language, yet each is only offering
—and receiving—a partial truth.

The patient, ashamed of past impulsivity or elevated moods,
minimizes them. The clinician, trained to prioritize present symptoms, may not probe deeply into the patient's history of energy shifts,
risk-taking, or episodic agitation. Each bias reinforces the other.
What emerges is not deception but a mutual mis-seeing.

Years may pass this way—years of incomplete diagnoses, partial
treatments, and recurrent crises. It can feel, in retrospect, as though
patient and clinician co-constructed the misunderstanding, not out
of negligence but out of the quiet collaboration of their biases. They

circled the truth without naming it, both guided by the limits of what felt speakable.

Wisdom interrupts this cycle. It reminds us to look again, to question the familiar story, to ask what has been underreported, overreported, or unconsciously disguised. It urges us to regard each clinical encounter not as a confirmation of prior patterns but as a new interpretive act, requiring curiosity and humility.

In this way, wisdom becomes the doorway through which diagnosis expands, treatment deepens, and suffering finally begins to make sense.

When Insight Arrives Slowly

A capable therapist sought treatment with me five years ago. She was already taking an antidepressant and reported feeling "fine."

After my initial evaluation and several follow-up visits, I gently suggested that she might do better on a mood stabilizer such as lamotrigine. Her response was polite but firm: she insisted she was well. Her clinical training, her identity as a therapist, and her fear of what a mood stabilizer might imply about her diagnosis created a subtle but powerful resistance. Her bias toward appearing competent met my bias toward diagnostic pattern recognition—and the stalemate held.

Four years later, during an unhurried session, she paused and admitted, "Maybe I do overthink and overreact—enough to cause distress for myself, my husband, and my children."

The sentence was quiet, but its meaning was vast. What she had minimized for years—emotional reactivity, rapid shifts in intensity, a lifelong pattern of internal escalation—finally rose into language.

She agreed to taper off the antidepressant and transition to a mood stabilizer. The difference was unmistakable. She felt steadier, more present, less consumed by internal storms. She enjoyed her family more. Work no longer demanded the constant emotional self-management she had assumed was normal.

Her improvement did not reveal a "missed" diagnosis—it revealed the power of slowly earned clarity. Her earlier refusal was not denial—it was self-protection shaped by professional identity, fear of stigma, and the quiet dread of what a different diagnosis might mean.

INTERPRETATION AS DESTINY

Nietzsche wrote that we live inside the interpretations we create—and often suffer inside the ones we inherit.

This patient had inherited an interpretation of herself as disciplined, emotionally controlled, endlessly resilient. Admitting instability felt like betrayal of that identity. Only when her interpretation expanded could her treatment expand.

In this sense, Nietzsche helps illuminate a central truth of clinical work: patients do not present symptoms—they present interpretations. And clinicians do not offer diagnoses—they offer counter-interpretations.

Where these two worlds of meaning collide, bias thrives. Where they meet with humility, something else becomes possible: transformation.

Wisdom is what allows both patient and clinician to revise their interpretations without shame—to let go of stories that once protected them but now confine them.

When this occurs, diagnosis deepens, treatment becomes more precise, and suffering begins, at last, to make sense.

∼

4

THE TRAGEDY OF
ABRUPT CONCLUSIONS

"Haste is universal because everyone is in flight from themselves."
— Friedrich Nietzsche

P sychiatry often operates under the illusion of linearity: a patient presents with symptoms, the clinician identifies a pattern, a diagnosis is made, and treatment begins. But human suffering is rarely linear. It is layered, recursive, shaped by forces that unfold over time. When clinicians reach conclusions too quickly—when they rush toward coherence rather than listening for complexity—they risk building entire treatment paths on foundations that cannot bear the weight of a patient's truth.

Abrupt conclusions do not arise from carelessness. They arise from pressure—internal, institutional, cultural—to produce clarity, to appear competent, to give patients something definitive to hold onto. Yet these premature answers can redirect a life, sometimes gently, sometimes decisively, away from what truly needs healing.

As Nietzsche warned, haste is not merely a behavioral impulse—

it is a psychic one. To rush is to avoid ourselves. Premature conclusions protect both patient and clinician from the discomfort of uncertainty. They create an illusion of clarity, masking deeper truths that require patience to uncover. Psychiatric misdiagnosis is often the result of fleeing complexity, not a lack of intelligence.

The Seduction of the First Explanation

There is a moment in every clinical encounter when the mind recognizes a pattern. A patient begins speaking and something familiar emerges. The clinician feels the pull of certainty: *I know this.* The diagnostic machinery activates. Symptoms align. Criteria fit. The case seems clear.

But the first explanation is often the most deceptive. It reflects what the patient is most prepared to disclose—and what the clinician is most prepared to hear. In this sense, both parties bring interpretations long before they bring truth.

A man once came to me with classic symptoms of panic disorder: racing heart, trembling, waves of terror. Several clinicians had previously confirmed this diagnosis. But when I asked him to describe the moments leading up to the episodes, he hesitated. The panic always struck when he was alone at night, thinking about a childhood he spent trying to make himself invisible.

His panic was not fear of losing control— it was the body's rebellion against decades of emotional silence. The diagnosis was not wrong, but it was incomplete. And incompleteness can mislead treatment as profoundly as error.

When Clinicians Mistake Clarity for Depth

Clarity is comforting. It offers shape to the formless and direction to uncertainty. But clarity reached too quickly, collapses complexity into something prematurely coherent.

A young woman came to me after years of treatment for bipolar disorder. She had been prescribed mood stabilizers, antipsychotics, and antidepressants. Some helped briefly; none helped deeply. Her mood chart showed fluctuations—but when we traced these fluctuations against the timeline of her relationships, a different picture emerged.

She did not have a mood disorder. She had a history of chronic invalidation—years of being told her feelings were "too much," her needs inconvenient. Her emotions rose and fell in response to attachment injury, not biology. Her episodes were protests against invisibility.

Her misdiagnosis did not arise from negligence. It arose from the clinician's desire to make sense of her quickly. Nietzsche would argue that humans cling to quick interpretations because uncertainty threatens the self. Psychiatry is not immune to this impulse.

THE HIDDEN COSTS of Premature Conclusions

When a clinician concludes too quickly, several things happen. The patient feels subtly unseen, even if treated with kindness. Treatment targets symptoms rather than meaning. Patients may blame themselves when treatment fails. Trust weakens; the therapeutic frame becomes brittle. And the true engine of suffering remains untouched.

Patients often internalize premature conclusions, living inside a story that never belonged to them. A man treated for depression may never discover the trauma beneath it. A woman treated for anxiety may never realize she is grieving. A teenager labeled "behavioral" may never have his loneliness named.

. . .

When Patients Adapt to Misunderstanding

Perhaps the most tragic outcome of abrupt conclusions is when patients mold themselves to match the clinician's initial interpretation. They reshape their narratives to remain legible. The clinical mistake becomes the shared reality.

A teenager once told me, after years of being labeled oppositional, "I guess I am difficult." But his difficulty was grief combined with fear—his father had left abruptly, and every time an adult raised their voice, he braced for abandonment. Opposition was a mask he wore to stay safe.

Had I accepted his initial story, he would have continued living inside a narrative that never reflected him.

The Patient Who Outgrew the Diagnosis Before the Clinician Did

A middle-aged man came to me with a seven-year history of "treatment-resistant depression." Multiple medications, several therapists, even a course of transcranial magnetic stimulation. His symptoms were consistent with depression.

But something in his narrative felt misaligned. His despair seemed situational, not biological. Mapping his episodes across life events revealed a pattern: he "became depressed" only during periods in which he was trapped in roles he had never chosen—caretaker, provider, mediator.

His despair was not endogenous. It was existential. He was living a life that violated his temperament. No one had slowed down enough to ask.

When we reframed his episodes as crises of authenticity rather than biochemical failure, everything changed. Therapy shifted toward agency, not symptoms. His so-called depression began to recede.

This is the silent harm of premature conclusions: when the right understanding arrives too late.

WISDOM as the Antidote to Haste

Wisdom slows the clinician's instinct to decide. It creates a pause in which deeper truth can surface.

Instead of asking *"What fits this picture?"* wisdom asks different questions: What am I missing? What else could this mean? What remains unspoken? What truth is the patient not yet strong enough to hold? How is my own training shaping what I see?

Wisdom replaces premature certainty with thoughtful curiosity. It tolerates ambiguity long enough for meaning to emerge.

THE LIFE-CHANGING Power of Slowness

The tragedy of abrupt conclusions lies not only in what they get wrong, but in what they obscure. Once a narrative takes hold, it resists revision.

But when clinicians slow down—listening for contradiction, attending to context, resisting seductive coherence—they give the patient something profoundly healing: the experience of being seen in depth.

Wisdom restores complexity. It protects patients from being reduced to their most visible suffering. It honors the slow, layered way the psyche reveals itself.

As Nietzsche reminds us, the deepest truths do not arrive through haste.

PART II

Seeing More Clearly

The symptom is never the whole story.

Part II moves beneath the surface — past language, past appearance, past the patient's own understanding of their suffering. Here, the clinician learns to perceive the emotional architecture that symptoms both reveal and conceal.

5

LISTENING BEYOND LANGUAGE

"What we hear is never all that is being said."
— Friedrich Nietzsche

Listening in psychiatry is far more than hearing words. It is an act of attunement—an interpretive art that gathers information from tone, pace, posture, silence, contradiction, and the emotional currents running beneath the surface of speech. People rarely say exactly what they mean. They say what feels safe, what feels possible, for what they have language.

Human speech conceals more than it reveals. The unsaid shapes the clinical encounter as strongly as the spoken. Wisdom listens beneath language, not merely to it.

A wise clinician listens not only to the story offered but to the one struggling to emerge.

Long before a patient forms a sentence, their body reveals the emotional landscape. A tightening of the jaw. A flicker of surprise. The way someone inhales sharply before admitting something painful. These subtle shifts tell truths that words have not yet caught up to.

A young man once told me in a steady voice that he felt "fine." But as he described his weakness, he pressed two fingers into his palm, leaving small crescents in his skin. His body contradicted his language. "Fine" was survival, not truth.

Listening beyond language means noticing the moments where the body disrupts the narrative.

SILENCE AS COMMUNICATION

Silence is not absence— it is information. It may signal fear, grief, shame, confusion, or a truth too fragile to touch. Many clinicians rush to fill silence to ease their own discomfort. But silence, when respected, allows meaning to rise.

A woman who had endured years of emotional neglect often fell silent when I asked about her childhood. I learned not to interpret this as resistance. Her silence was the closest she could come to remembering.

Wisdom hears the weight of what cannot yet be spoken.

WHEN WORDS and Emotion Diverge

A patient's emotional tone is often a truer guide than their narrative. When the feeling in the room contradicts the words being spoken, the clinician must pause.

A man once described his anxiety in a detached, almost cheerful voice. But the room felt tight, breathless. His emotional tone belonged to fear. His voice belonged to denial.

The wise clinician asks: Which truth is this patient able to show, and which truth must they hide?

Cultural Languages, Emotional Languages

Not all cultures communicate distress directly. Some use metaphor. Some use idioms. Some use the body. Some use silence. Listening beyond language requires humility—recognizing that what sounds like avoidance in one culture may be token of respect in another.

A clinician who listens only for Western emotional vocabulary will miss vast regions of the patient's world.

The Music of Speech

Every patient carries a rhythm—pauses, hesitations, repeated phrases, rising or falling intonations. These elements reveal emotional truths that the content alone cannot.

Some people speak in circles because their story is too overwhelming to approach directly. Others speak too quickly because they fear they will lose courage if they slow down. Others repeat themselves because they are waiting to see if the clinician finally hears the meaning behind the words.

Listening With the Whole Self

To listen beyond language, the clinician must bring emotional openness, suspension of judgment, sensitivity to contradiction, comfort with silence, and awareness of their own internal reactions.

Often, what the clinician feels in the room—anxiety, heaviness, sadness—is a clue to what the patient cannot express.

Listening beyond language transforms the encounter. It turns the clinical hour into a shared space where truth can surface, even when words fail.

LISTENING When Language Barely Exists

Some of the deepest lessons about listening came from working with very young children— three-year-olds whose suffering had not yet acquired words. Their speech was limited, but their bodies spoke urgently: arched backs, trembling hands, darting eyes, sudden stillness, or explosive tears. The child's body became the primary narrator, the parents' stories the secondary, and my task was to listen to both without assuming that either was complete.

In these encounters, I learned that aggression in a toddler often disguised terror, that withdrawal was sometimes the only safe strategy a young child had, that a tantrum could be a primitive plea for regulation rather than defiance. The parents' distress was equally revealing—guilt, exhaustion, fear of judgment, and the heavy cultural belief that children this young should not have serious emotional problems. Many hesitated to acknowledge the severity of the symptoms because doing so opened the door to interventions they feared, particularly the possibility of medication.

Listening beyond language in early childhood care meant attending to sequences. What preceded the scream? What followed the stillness? When did fear enter the room? The child's body and the family's narrative formed a fragile duet, each exposing what the other concealed.

Often, only after an atmosphere of deep empathy was established did parents reveal the full picture—the nighttime terrors, the sudden freezes, the inexplicable dread around certain people or places. Their hesitation was not deception but fear: fear of stigma, fear of being seen as inadequate, fear that naming the truth would unleash interventions they were not ready to face.

In those moments, I understood Nietzsche's reminder that the greatest part of what we know is unwanted, and we keep it hidden until we can bear it. Young children cannot hide in words, but adults hide on their behalf—until the clinician creates enough safety for the truth to surface.

Listening beyond language here required something more elemental than skill: the willingness to inhabit the child's pre-verbal world and honor the family's fear without letting it obscure the child's reality.

~

6

DEPTH PERCEPTION IN PSYCHIATRY

"The depths are not reached by a single plunge."
— Friedrich Nietzsche

Depth perception in psychiatry is the ability to see the layered terrain of a patient's emotional life—where symptoms are surface weather and the true climate lies underground. Most human suffering does not announce itself directly. It lives in the folds of memory, in inherited narratives, in old adaptations that have outlived their usefulness. Yet clinicians are often trained to work at the surface, to treat symptoms as destinations rather than signals.

Depth reveals truths that symptoms alone cannot show. Healing requires descending slowly into layers the patient cannot reach alone. Wisdom grows only when the clinician resists the illusion of the surface.

Depth perception widens the clinician's gaze from the immediate complaint to the long arc of a life. It asks not only *What is happening now?* but *What has been happening for years?*

THE VERTICAL DIMENSION

Symptoms emerge from timelines—often long, often invisible. Depression in adulthood may be the echo of childhood silences. Panic may rise from years spent anticipating danger. Identity conflict may bloom where cultural and personal worlds collide.

Nietzsche wrote that the depths are not reached by a single plunge. Human psychology is the same: depth requires descending slowly, layer by layer, with humility.

Wisdom invites the clinician to follow the symptom downward—to its origins, its evolution, its emotional meaning.

STATE VS. TRAIT

One of psychiatry's most essential distinctions is between what is state-based and what is trait-based. States shift with circumstance; they reflect the present. Traits persist over time; they shape the emotional architecture of a life.

Mistaking a trait for a state creates false hope. Mistaking a state for a trait creates unnecessary despair.

A woman once came to me grieving a divorce. Her hopelessness resembled depression, but her history carried no depressive pattern. Her sorrow was not a flaw in her biology—it was grief searching for its place.

Depth perception guards against conclusions that collapse a moment into an identity.

· · ·

THE INFLUENCE of Emotional History

Every present emotion carries the weight of earlier ones. People reenact patterns learned before they could speak. They carry voices that are not their own. They respond to today with strategies forged decades earlier.

A man who had been criticized throughout childhood answered every question with caution. His voice had learned to whisper. Without depth perception, his hesitancy might have been misdiagnosed as anxiety. With depth, it became clear: he was still bracing for the reprimands of a past that lived inside him.

Nietzsche observed that we become the heirs of our unlived lives. Emotional history is not simply remembered—it is enacted.

CONTEXT AS COMPASS

Depth perception requires attention to context: family narratives, cultural identity, developmental turning points, social roles and expectations, trauma memory, and attachment patterns.

Context transforms a symptom into a story—and a story into understanding.

SEEING the Layers at Once

Depth perception is multidimensional. A single symptom may arise from several emotional strata simultaneously: unprocessed grief, cultural restriction, fear of abandonment, trauma residue, identity conflict. The wise clinician listens for the dominant emotional layer without erasing the others.

A young man described irritability that seemed purely behavioral. But when we explored further, his irritability was a shield—

protecting him from the terror of being left. Beneath the anger lived a small boy who had once been abandoned.

The Architecture Beneath the Symptom

A teenager was referred for "defiance." His teachers saw disruption; his parents saw disrespect. But during our sessions, he flinched whenever I raised my voice even slightly. Over time, he revealed that as a child, every mistake was met with disproportionate punishment. His "defiance" was an old survival strategy—stay distant, stay guarded, stay unpredictable so no one can corner you.

Had I treated only the behavior, I would have missed the fear that shaped it.

Depth perception exposes the architecture beneath the symptom.

Depth as a Path to Healing

People heal not when symptoms vanish, but when their suffering is understood in full context. Depth perception allows the clinician to see the entire emotional landscape—the long seasons of a life, not merely the present weather.

When patients feel seen in depth, something within them settles. They sense that their story is held not as a collection of problems but as a coherent, complicated whole.

Depth perception turns the clinical encounter from an interview into a revelation—an unveiling of the person beneath the symptom.

~

7

HOLDING CONTRADICTIONS

"We are both the marble and the sculptor."
— Friedrich Nietzsche

Human beings are contradictory by nature. We want closeness and fear it. We crave change and resist it. We long to be understood yet hide the truths that would allow anyone to know us. Contradiction is not evidence of pathology —it is the emotional tension through which a life organizes itself.

Contradiction is the medium through which the self-shapes itself. Emotional conflict reveals truth, not disorder. Meaning emerges where opposing forces meet.

Clinicians who seek neat coherence often mistake to see contradiction for instability, inconsistency, or manipulation. But wisdom teaches that contradiction is a diagnostic clue, not a clinical obstacle.

CONTRADICTIONS REVEAL Emotional Truths

A woman once told me she wanted desperately to leave a destructive relationship—yet she could not imagine life without the person harming her. This was not ambivalence. It was attachment wrestling with survival, longing wrapped around fear.

Contradiction exposes the internal conflict that symptoms can only gesture toward.

Nietzsche wrote that we are both the marble and the sculptor, suggesting that humans are shaped by opposing forces within themselves. In psychiatry, contradiction is where those forces meet.

COHERENCE IS OFTEN the Enemy of Truth

When clinicians demand coherence, patients begin to edit their truth to appear consistent. They simplify themselves to avoid seeming confused. They smooth their story to protect the clinician's approval.

But contradictions carry essential emotional truths: love mixed with resentment, longing mixed with fear, hope mixed with shame, anger mixed with grief.

To insist on coherence is to flatten the emotional landscape.

THE CLINICIAN'S Discomfort With Ambiguity

Contradiction unsettles clinicians because it disrupts certainty. We are taught to categorize, to decide, to resolve. But resolution reached too early could be a form of erasure.

A teenager once told me he hated his mother and wanted to protect her at the same time. A clinician before me labeled this "manipulation." But it was trauma bonding— love fused to fear through years of unpredictable caregiving.

Contradiction was not the problem. It was the map.

. . .

The Doorway to Emotional Architecture

A young man came to me describing intense social anxiety. Yet he also described a desire to perform on stage, to be seen, to be recognized. His previous clinician viewed this as inconsistency.

But when we explored further, the contradiction revealed an identity split formed in childhood—celebrated for achievement, punished for emotion. He longed to be visible but feared the vulnerability visibility required.

Contradiction was the doorway to understanding the emotional architecture beneath his symptoms.

Holding Contradictions Without Resolving Them

Wise clinicians do not rush to resolve contradictions. They hold them gently, creating space for the patient to explore emotional tensions without shame or pressure.

Holding contradiction requires emotional patience, suspension of judgment, recognition of context, and comfort with complexity.

The goal is not to choose one truth but to understand why both truths exist.

The Transformative Power of Being Understood in Complexity

When a patient realizes that they do not need to simplify themselves to be taken seriously, something fundamental shifts. Shame softens. Defenses loosen. Grief begins to articulate itself.

Contradiction becomes a site of expansion. Instead of being asked to collapse into clarity, the patient is invited to inhabit the full range of their emotional experience.

Wisdom holds what logic cannot.

THE SIGNATURE of Being Human

Logic seeks clarity. Wisdom seeks wholeness. And wholeness includes conflict.

To understand a person is to understand their contradictions—not as errors, but as expressions of their emotional truth.

Contradiction is not a failure of coherence. It is the signature of being human.

∾

8

SEEING BEYOND SYMPTOMS

"We are obliged to see surfaces first."
— Friedrich Nietzsche

Symptoms are only the surface of suffering—a thin crust covering a much deeper terrain. They shimmer with fragments of truth, but they are not the truth itself. To rely on symptoms alone is to mistake the reflection for the source, the shadow for the body that casts it. Modern psychiatry, in its desire for clarity and efficiency, often treats symptoms as primary facts. But symptoms are merely the language suffering uses when it has no other means to speak.

To see beyond symptoms is to listen past what is obvious, past what is rehearsed, past what fits neatly into diagnostic categories. It is to recognize that every symptom is a messenger from somewhere deeper.

As Nietzsche observed, we are obliged to see surfaces first. This is the human condition: we cling to what is visible, what is nameable, what is measurable—even when the real story lies somewhere the eye cannot immediately reach. Wisdom begins the moment we stop mistaking surface for essence.

THE TEMPTATION of Symptom-Centered Thinking

Symptom-centered thinking offers the comfort of decisiveness. Checklists bring order. Criteria sharpen conclusions. Treatment pathways appear straightforward. But this clarity can seduce the clinician into a form of tunnel vision.

A young man once told me he felt "low energy," "foggy," and "unmotivated." Classic signs of depression, perhaps even hypothyroidism, or burnout. But something in the flat way he recited the symptoms felt too distant from true anguish. When I asked him what had changed in his life, he shrugged. Only later did he confess that he had abandoned his passion for music after years of familial ridicule.

His symptoms were not defects. They were grief in disguise.

Symptoms describe how a person suffers— not why.

CONTEXT as the Missing Diagnostic Dimension

No symptom exists in isolation. It lives inside a web of relationships, buried histories, identity tensions, cultural scripts, and long-standing emotional demands.

Depression in a teenager wrestling with identity is different from depression in a parent carrying invisible burdens. Anxiety in a child of immigrants means something different than anxiety in a retired man facing mortality. The same symptom can emerge from trauma, biology, chronic loneliness, cultural conflict, or moral injury.

Without context, even an accurate diagnosis can miss the emotional truth.

Nietzsche reminds us that meaning is not discovered—it is constructed. Symptoms acquire meaning only when placed inside the story of a life.

The Deep Structure of Suffering

To see beyond symptoms is to attune to what lies beneath: the origin of the symptom, the function it serves, the emotional meaning it carries, the cultural script shaping its expression, the developmental history that formed it, and the identity conflict it may be protecting.

A patient once reported intense social anxiety. On the surface: fear of judgment, fear of speaking, fear of exposure. But when we traced the anxiety back through her past, a deeper truth emerged. She had been told all her life that she was "too much", too emotional, too expressive, too alive. Her anxiety was not about people. It was about the terror of being seen.

Her symptom was the echo of a childhood wound.

When Symptoms Protect More Than They Distress

Some symptoms are not alarms—they are shields.

A man with chronic irritability appeared volatile, oppositional, quick to anger. But when we slowed down and explored carefully, a different picture unfolded. His irritability was the only emotion that had ever been permitted in his home. Vulnerability had always been punished. Anger was his armor.

To treat irritability directly would have stripped him of his only protection without addressing the fear beneath it.

Wisdom sees symptoms not as enemies to eliminate but as survival strategies written into the psyche.

THE WOMAN WHO "COULDN'T FOCUS"

A woman in her thirties was referred to me for suspected ADHD. She described distractibility, difficulty completing tasks, mental drifting. On paper, the symptoms matched. But when I asked when these difficulties first began, her eyes fell to the floor.

"After my divorce," she said quietly.

As we explored further, it became clear that her mind was not scattered— it was grieving. Her inattention was a form of protest, a refusal to engage fully with a life that had become emotionally unrecognizable.

She was not losing focus. She was losing the world she had built.

Her symptom was not indicative of disorder. It was sorrow asking to be acknowledged.

SEEING in Layers

To see beyond symptoms is to perceive the layers of experience from which they arise. It requires the clinician to slow down, to ask questions that invite depth rather than speed, to notice contradictions and emotional dissonance, to treat emotion as data, and to listen for the story beneath the story.

Symptoms open the door—but wisdom walks through it.

LOOKING THROUGH, Not At

To treat only the symptom is to aim at the reflection on the surface of the water. To understand the suffering beneath is to reach the source.

Symptoms are the first language of distress. But they are not the final truth.

The wise clinician resists the seduction of visibility. They look through symptoms, not at them. They understand that what is most important is often what the symptom protects, obscures, or represents.

And when we learn to see in this way—slowly, deeply, with humility—we begin to treat not the shadow, but the person who casts it.

∼

PART III

When Diagnosis Is Not Enough

Accuracy without attunement is not yet healing.

Even correct diagnoses fail when they ignore meaning, timing, shame, and readiness. Part III confronts the hidden reasons treatment falters — and shows why the person must be understood alongside the condition.

9

THE HIT-AND-MISS REALITY
OF MODERN TREATMENT

"We are complicated beings; a single truth rarely explains us."
— Friedrich Nietzsche

Modern psychiatric treatment is often described as if it were a precise science: diagnose correctly, choose the evidence-based intervention, apply it diligently, and the patient improves. This narrative comforts clinicians and reassures the public. But the lived reality of treatment is far messier— shaped by personality, culture, ambivalence, identity, shame, trauma, and the patient's own conflict about change.

Psychiatric outcomes cannot be predicted by diagnosis alone. Even accurate labels fail to capture the emotional conflicts that shape healing. People respond not to treatments in general, but to treatments as they collide with their histories, identities, and fears.

Treatment succeeds and fails for reasons far deeper than diagnosis alone. Even when we name the condition accurately, we may still miss the human being who lives inside it.

· · ·

Correct Diagnosis, Missed Meaning

A patient may receive the right diagnosis yet make little or no progress. This frustrates clinicians and devastates patients. But diagnosis, while necessary, is not sufficient.

A man with major depression may fail multiple medications because his suffering is rooted not in neurochemistry but in ungrieved loss. A woman with social anxiety may improve only marginally with exposure therapy because her avoidance is driven not by fear of people but by a shame narrative inherited in childhood.

Treatment fails when we treat symptoms instead of meaning.

The Emotional Weight of Diagnosis

Patients do not receive diagnoses as neutral pieces of information. A diagnosis is an emotional event. It can validate or shame, frighten or liberate, confirm hidden fears, or reshape identity, alter family narratives, or crystallize a new understanding of the self.

A young woman burst into tears when told she had ADHD—tears of relief. For the first time, her lifelong struggles made sense. Another patient, given the exact same diagnosis, froze. To him, it felt like confirmation of every hurtful label he had internalized since childhood.

The same diagnosis can heal or harm depending on the story into which it falls.

Why Evidence-Based Treatments Often Miss

Evidence-based treatments are essential. But they are built on group averages, not individual lives. They quietly assume stable motivation, consistent insight, emotional readiness, cultural neutrality, and a patient who feels deserving of care. Most patients do not arrive with these prerequisites.

A woman once failed two rounds of cognitive behavioral therapy for depression and was labeled "treatment resistant." Yet when we explored her history, we discovered her entire identity was built around self-sacrifice. The directive to prioritize herself triggered overwhelming guilt.

She was not resistant— she was conflicted.

Treatment succeeded only when we addressed guilt, not the thoughts.

Personal Factors That Shift Outcomes

Treatment outcomes depend on variables that no protocol can fully capture trust in the clinician, cultural beliefs about suffering, family expectations, internalized shame, readiness for change, emotional literacy, stability of identity, and relational patterns.

A patient may refuse medication not because they doubt its usefulness, but because "needing it" feels like moral failure within their cultural or familial world.

The Myth of Linear Improvement

Most people imagine healing as a steady ascent. But the true pattern is nonlinear—alive, unpredictable, and human. Two steps forward, one step back. Long plateaus. Sudden regressions. Breakthroughs triggered by unrelated events. Emotional growth appears only in retrospect.

Regression is not failure—it is part of the psyche's attempt to reorganize.

.   .   .

When Treatment Works Despite Imperfection

Remarkably, treatment often succeeds even when imperfectly matched—if the therapeutic relationship is strong. Patients heal not because the intervention itself is flawless, but because they feel understood.

A protocol is a map. Relationship is terrain.

Wisdom recognizes that treatment is not mechanical. It is interpretive, relational, and deeply human— shaped by timing, trust, meaning, and the patient's readiness to encounter their own truth.

Modern treatment is hit and miss because human beings do not heal by formula. They heal through understanding, connection, and the slow, unfolding work of being truly seen.

10

DENIAL, SHAME, AND
THE SOCIAL MIRROR

"We remain unknown to ourselves."
— Friedrich Nietzsche

Denial is not blindness—it is a form of inner architecture. People do not turn away from truth because they are stubborn or careless. They turn away because some truths arrive like earthquakes: too destabilizing, too identity-threatening, too incompatible with the stories that have protected them for years. Shame works similarly—not as a mere emotion, but as a governing force that polices visibility. It decides what one may know about oneself, and what one may allow others to witness.

Denial is protection from truths that feel too destabilizing to face. Shame governs what may be revealed—and what must remain hidden—even from oneself. Self-knowledge emerges only when the mind becomes strong enough to tolerate what it once avoided.

Modern psychiatry often treats denial and shame as obstacles to treatment. Wisdom sees them as survival strategies— ingenious, adaptive, and deeply human. They must be understood before they are loosened.

Nietzsche wrote that we remain unknown to ourselves, not because self-knowledge is impossible, but because we defend ourselves against truths that might undo us. Denial and shame are two of the primary defenses.

DENIAL as Emotional Architecture

People do not deny facts; they deny meanings. A man who refuses to acknowledge his drinking problem is not denying the alcohol. He is denying what it would mean to be "a failure," "like his father," or "someone who needs help." Denial protects identity. It shields the self from collapse.

A woman once insisted she was not depressed despite every symptom pointing to the contrary. Her home immaculate, her schedule precise, her emotions perfectly contained— her ordered world was her fortress. Depression threatened the identity she had crafted to survive a chaotic childhood. To admit suffering would mean admitting vulnerability. Denial was her scaffolding.

Even the simple act of coming to a psychiatrist carries its own hierarchy of denial: *I am here, but perhaps it's not that bad; I need help, but maybe not that kind.* Diagnosis, treatment options, even medication choices all become weighed against a private scale of what the patient can bear to acknowledge.

SHAME as a Social Emotion

Shame is born in an imagined audience. It is relational through and through. It arises in anticipation of how one might be seen—by family, community, culture, or clinician.

A teenager withheld his panic attacks because he feared appearing "weak." A retired man minimized his suicidal thoughts because in his culture, suffering signaled personal failure. Shame distorts reporting, delays diagnosis, and can bend the entire arc of treatment.

But shame is also diagnostic. It points directly to where a patient feels least worthy, least protected.

THE SOCIAL MIRROR

People see themselves not only through their own eyes but through the gaze they expect from their world. A diagnosis that feels neutral to a clinician may feel catastrophic to a patient if it threatens their standing in their family or community.

A young woman feared starting therapy because in her family, seeking help meant disloyalty—a sign that the family had failed. Another patient resisted medication because in his community, needing help was equated with moral weakness.

To understand a patient, one must understand the social mirror through which they view themselves.

WHEN DENIAL Is Mistaken for Resistance

Clinicians often misinterpret denial as stubbornness, avoidance, or opposition. But denial is seldom about the clinician. It is about what acknowledgment might unleash.

A man who had lost his job insisted he was "fine." To admit devastation would mean confronting the fragility of a self-worth built entirely on achievement. Treatment began only when we addressed the meaning of failure—not the symptoms of depression.

Nietzsche noted that humans prefer the familiar unhappiness to an unfamiliar truth. Denial is the psyche's way of preserving the familiar.

Working With Denial, Not Against It

Wisdom does not attack denial. It respects the purpose denial serves and gently expands the patient's capacity to know.

This involves slowing the pace of insight, creating psychological safety, naming emotions without shame, validating survival strategies, and allowing truth to surface gradually.

Denial dissolves when the patient becomes strong enough to face what was once unbearable.

Shame as a Barrier to Healing

Shame hides the very emotions that need tending. Patients avoid discussing trauma, dependency, rage, envy, or neediness because these contradict the identities they have been taught to uphold.

A clinician who listens without judgment disarms shame simply by remaining present. When shame loses its secrecy, healing begins.

How Denial and Shame Shape Treatment Trajectories

Denial and shame shape not only what patients say but how they engage with treatment.

Some arrive eager, then vanish when conversation nears a forbidden truth. Others attend consistently but remain emotionally motionless. Still others improve briefly, then regress when growth threatens a role that has anchored their identity.

A lifelong caregiver may unconsciously sabotage progress if healing threatens the role that gives her purpose. A man whose survival depended on emotional invisibility may retreat when therapy asks him to develop a voice.

Denial and shame are not barriers. They are coordinates—they show us where the psyche feels endangered.

Helping Patients Reclaim Disowned Parts

Healing often requires welcoming back the emotions a patient deemed unacceptable: grief that once felt disloyal, anger that once felt dangerous, neediness that once felt shameful, vulnerability that once felt weak.

When these emotions re-enter the patient's world without judgment, identity expands. Denial loosens. Shame thins. The psyche becomes more spacious.

The Gentle Unmasking of Truth

Denial and shame are not pathologies— they are protections. Wisdom does not strip these protections away. It helps patients outgrow them.

When that happens, truth does not crash in. It arrives quietly, like something long known finally permitted to speak.

This is the quiet miracle of psychiatric healing: the slow emergence of a self that is no longer defined by what it must hide.

~

11

THE DROPOUT PHENOMENON

"We flee not from suffering, but from the meanings we cannot bear."
— Friedrich Nietzsche

P atients rarely leave treatment because they no longer need help. More often, they leave because therapy has approached a truth they cannot yet bear. Dropout is not abandonment. It is communication— a message sent through disappearance.

Dropout is rarely about avoidance. It is about escaping a truth that feels too destabilizing. Patients often leave precisely when therapy approaches an emotional fault line. Meaning, not symptoms, is what threatens the psyche most deeply.

Nietzsche observed that human beings flee not from suffering, but from the meanings they cannot tolerate. Dropout is often precisely this: a flight from meaning.

. . .

WHY PATIENTS VANISH

Patients disengage when therapy draws too close to truths that threaten identity, emotions they were never permitted to feel, shame that has begun to surface, family or cultural narratives they fear challenging, the possibility of disappointing the clinician, memories that feel too dangerous to name, or changes that destabilize long-held roles.

A man once stopped therapy abruptly after weeks of progress. Months later he confessed, "You were seeing too much." His departure was not avoidance but self-preservation.

THE EMOTIONAL LOGIC of Leaving

Leaving treatment often reflects fear of vulnerability, fear of dependence, fear of collapsing if the truth is spoken, dread of confirming a diagnosis already feared, or the belief that one is "too much" or "not fixable."

People do not flee therapy. They flee what therapy makes visible.

A young woman who survived chronic invalidation once disappeared from treatment the moment she began to articulate anger. For her, anger had always been punished. The emergence of that feeling triggered the ancient fear of being emotionally annihilated.

CLINICIAN Misinterpretations

Clinicians may misread dropout as resistance, lack of motivation, disorganization, or noncompliance. But wisdom asks a different set of questions. What was the patient protecting by leaving? What rose too quickly? What became too close to truth?

Nietzsche warned about the danger of premature illumination—

truth arriving faster than the psyche can metabolize. Dropout is often the psyche dimming the light to survive.

THE DISAPPEARING ADOLESCENT

A teenager began therapy for depression. After a breakthrough session exploring his loneliness, he vanished. When he returned two months later, he said: "I didn't want you to know how much it mattered."

His disappearance was an attempt to regain emotional control.

Dropout often appears where attachment and fear meet.

RE-ENGAGEMENT WITHOUT BLAME

When patients return, the wise clinician welcomes them without disappointment or punitive curiosity. Return is an act of courage— a sign that the patient is ready to approach the truth again, but at a different pace.

Dropout is the psyche's way of pacing the work.

⟅⟆

12

THE LIMITS OF PROTOCOLS

"All great things must first wear a mask."
— Friedrich Nietzsche

P rotocols are invaluable—they organize knowledge, create consistency, and guide clinical action. But they are designed for patterns, not for people. They capture what is statistically effective, not what is emotionally possible.

Protocols can see symptoms. They cannot see context.

Symptoms often disguise their origins, and protocols mistake the mask for the truth. Protocols treat patterns, while wisdom must treat people. What appears clinically clear often conceals a deeper emotional reality.

Nietzsche wrote that all great things must first wear a mask. Symptoms often wear the mask of clarity; protocols mistake the mask for the person.

.   .   .

The Checklist Fallacy

Protocols assume stable motivation, consistent emotional capacity, culturally neutral expressions of distress, and readiness for cognitive or behavioral change. But human beings do not move in straight lines. They regress, recoil, surge forward, collapse, and rebuild.

A woman with PTSD once struggled intensely with trauma-focused therapy. Protocol advised continuing. Wisdom advised pausing. Her nervous system was not yet prepared for exposure.

The intervention was correct; the timing was not.

Protocols name the path. Wisdom discerns the pace.

When Protocols Cannot See Context

Protocols cannot account for cultural prohibitions against disclosure, family loyalty conflicts, identity crisis, shame dynamics, attachment wounds, trauma-shaped expectations of danger, or emotional skill deficits.

A teenager "failed" exposure therapy for social anxiety. He wasn't avoidant—he simply couldn't name his fear. He needed safety first, then language, before facing exposure.

A correct treatment delivered too early becomes incorrect.

When Protocols Work Against Healing

Some protocols push patients into emotional territory they are not yet able to navigate. Others focus on cognition when the patient is drowning in shame. Still others assume insight where none exists.

A man with panic disorder failed multiple treatment modalities until someone finally noticed that every panic episode followed calls from his estranged mother. His panic was not a biological glitch—it was an attachment alarm.

. . .

Adapting Protocols Rather Than Abandoning Them

The critique of protocols is not a call to discard them. Protocols represent hard-won knowledge—decades of research distilled into actionable guidance. The problem arises when protocols are applied rigidly, as though the map were the territory, as though the average patient in a study were the specific person sitting in the room.

Wisdom does not abandon protocols. It inhabits them differently.

Adaptation begins with sequencing. A protocol may be entirely appropriate for a patient—but not yet. A woman with obsessive-compulsive disorder may benefit enormously from exposure and response prevention, but if she arrives in a state of chronic hyper-arousal, with no internal sense of safety, exposure will feel like re-traumatization rather than treatment. The wise clinician builds the foundation first: nervous system regulation, therapeutic trust, and emotional vocabulary. The protocol remains the destination, but the path to it must be cleared.

Adaptation also involves pacing. Protocols often assume a rhythm of progress that real patients cannot sustain. A man working through trauma-focused cognitive behavioral therapy may need to slow down after a particularly destabilizing session—not because he is resistant, but because integration takes time. Wisdom reads the patient's capacity session by session, adjusting intensity the way a skilled teacher adjusts the difficulty of material to match the learner's readiness.

Adaptation requires attention to meaning. The same intervention can land differently depending on how it is framed. A behavioral activation protocol for depression asks patients to schedule pleasurable activities. For some, this is liberating. For others—particularly those whose depression is rooted in a lifetime of self-denial—it triggers guilt or shame. The wise clinician does not abandon the intervention; instead, they address the meaning first. Why does pleasure feel forbidden? What old voice says you do not deserve relief? Once the meaning is metabolized, the protocol becomes usable.

Adaptation demands cultural humility. Protocols developed in one cultural context may require significant modification in another. Exposure therapy for social anxiety assumes that avoidance is the problem and approach is the solution. But for a patient whose culture values restraint, modesty, or deference to authority, "approach" may need to be redefined. The goal is not to impose a Western model of social confidence but to help the patient move toward their own values with less suffering. The protocol bends to meet the person.

Adaptation also means knowing when to set a protocol aside temporarily. Sometimes a patient arrives in crisis, and the structured work must pause. Sometimes an unexpected disclosure reshapes the entire treatment. Sometimes the therapeutic relationship itself becomes the intervention, and no manual can guide what unfolds. In these moments, the clinician holds the protocol lightly, returning to it when the patient is ready.

The adapted protocol is not a weakened protocol. It is a protocol made wise— fitted to the contours of a particular life, delivered at a pace the psyche can absorb, framed in language that honors the patient's world. Research gives us the "what". Wisdom gives us the when, the how, and the why it matters to this person.

Protocols are tools. Wisdom is the hand that wields them.

WISDOM ADAPTS Where Protocols End

Wisdom is not anti-science. It is what renders science humane.

Protocols emerge from controlled conditions—randomized trials, manualized treatments, carefully selected participants, measurable outcomes. These conditions are necessary for generating reliable knowledge. But the consulting room is not a controlled condition. It is a living encounter between two people, shaped by history, culture, emotion, and the unpredictable movements of trust.

Wisdom begins when the protocol falls silent. It asks questions that no manual can answer. What does this patient need right now— not in general, but in this moment, on this day, given what has just surfaced? What emotional scaffolding must be built before the structured work can begin? What truth is this symptom protecting, and what would happen if we approached it too quickly? What would it mean to slow down, to wait, to let the patient set the pace?

These are not questions of technique. They are questions of attunement.

Wisdom also holds what protocols cannot name: the therapeutic relationship itself. Research consistently shows that the quality of the alliance between clinician and patient predicts outcomes more reliably than the specific modality employed. A patient may receive the most evidence-based treatment available and still fail to improve if they do not feel seen, understood, or safe. Conversely, a patient may heal through a treatment that is theoretically imperfect but delivered by a clinician who listens deeply and responds with care.

This does not mean that relationship replaces technique. It means that relationship is the medium through which technique becomes tolerable. A protocol is a set of instructions. Wisdom is the presence that makes those instructions bearable.

Wisdom also recognizes that healing is not always linear or legible. Protocols measure progress through symptom reduction, behavioral change, or functional improvement. These are valid metrics. But some of the most important movements in treatment leave no trace on a checklist. A patient who finally allows herself to cry in session has crossed a threshold that no scale can capture. A man who admits, for the first time, that he is afraid has begun a process that may take years to unfold. Wisdom honors these invisible shifts, holding them as evidence of change even when the protocol sees stagnation.

There are also moments when wisdom requires setting the protocol aside entirely—not out of negligence, but out of respect for what is emerging. A patient in the middle of structured trauma work may disclose something unexpected: a new memory, a relational crisis, a sudden wave of grief unrelated to the treatment focus. The protocol would say to return to the agenda. Wisdom may say to stay with what has arrived. These are clinical judgments that cannot be scripted. They require a clinician who is present, flexible, and willing to tolerate uncertainty.

Wisdom does not reject the knowledge that protocols contain. It contextualizes that knowledge within a larger understanding of what it means to help a suffering person. It asks not only "What does the evidence say?" but also "What does this person need in order to receive what the evidence offers?" The answer is almost always the same: they need to feel safe, to feel seen, and to feel that the clinician is with them rather than ahead of them.

Protocols guide treatment. They offer structure, direction, and accountability. They protect patients from idiosyncratic or harmful interventions. They represent the collective wisdom of the field, refined through decades of inquiry.

But protocols cannot hold a patient's hand when terror rises. They cannot sit in silence when words fail. They cannot recognize the moment when a patient is ready to know something they have spent a lifetime avoiding. They cannot feel the shift in the room when trust finally takes root.

Wisdom does these things. Wisdom is what remains when the manual has nothing left to say.

Protocols guide treatment. Wisdom guides healing.

PART IV

Toward a Wiser Psychiatry

From understanding to presence. From presence to healing.

Part IV traces the movement from clinical skill to clinical wisdom.
Here, psychiatry becomes something more than diagnosis and
prescription. It becomes accompaniment — the quiet, steady work of
helping patients revise lives they once believed were fixed.

13

WHAT CLINICAL WISDOM
LOOKS LIKE IN PRACTICE

"There is no truth, only perspectives."
— Friedrich Nietzsche

W isdom in psychiatry is not mystical. It is practical, observable, and profoundly relational. It arises when the clinician integrates emotion, context, perception, and humility.

Wisdom begins where single- perspective thinking ends. Psychiatry becomes most healing when it welcomes complexity rather than resolves it. Clinicians and patients both arrive with interpretations—wisdom integrates them.

The Six Pillars of Clinical Wisdom

Clinical wisdom rests on capacities that can be named, cultivated, and recognized in practice.

The first is meta-perception: seeing how the patient sees themselves. Wisdom requires understanding not only what the patient feels but how they understand their own feeling. Most suffering comes partly from the emotion itself, and partly from how the patient interprets it. A man who feels sadness and believes it means he is weak suffers twice—once from the sadness, once from the self-judgment. The wise clinician attends to both the layers.

The second is emotional integration: using one's own emotional responses as data. The clinician's internal reactions—heaviness, agitation, warmth, confusion—are often signals the patient cannot yet articulate. When a clinician feels inexplicably drained after a session, or strangely protective, or subtly irritated, these responses deserve attention. They may be pointing toward something the patient has not yet spoken.

The third is perspective taking: holding multiple possible truths at once. A wise clinician resists collapsing complexity into a single, clean explanation. A patient's anger may be justified and destructive, their grief appropriate and prolonged, their avoidance protective and limiting. Wisdom holds these tensions without rushing to resolve them.

The fourth is uncertainty tolerance: resisting premature conclusions. Certainty feels good; it is rarely accurate. Wisdom slows the impulse to "know." It sits with ambiguity long enough for deeper patterns to emerge, recognizing that the first formulation is often incomplete.

The fifth is proportionality: matching interpretation to context and severity. Not every sadness is depression. Not every panic is anxiety. Not every silence is avoidance. Wisdom calibrates, distinguishing between a life crisis and a clinical disorder, between a developmental struggle and a chronic condition, between suffering that requires intervention and suffering that requires witness.

The sixth is moral orientation: grounding decisions in compassion and dignity. Wisdom protects the patient's humanity, especially when they cannot protect theirs. It refuses to reduce a person to their symptoms, their failures, or their worst moments. It holds the patient as someone deserving of care, even when they cannot believe this about themselves.

These six pillars do not operate in isolation. In any given session, they interweave— the clinician reading the patient's self-perception, noticing their own emotional response, holding multiple interpretations, tolerating uncertainty, calibrating severity, and orienting toward the patient's dignity. Wisdom is not a single capacity but a constellation of capacities working together.

THE WISE SESSION

A wise session is not dramatic. It is spacious.

It allows patients to contradict themselves without being corrected, to hesitate without being hurried, to grieve without being reassured too quickly, to express anger without consequence, to revise old narratives without shame, and to speak without fear of misunderstanding.

The wise clinician does not fill every silence. They do not interpret every pause. They do not steer the conversation toward what they expect to find. They create room for the unexpected, for the half-formed thought, for the emotion that has no name yet.

Wisdom creates the conditions in which truth becomes possible.

A YOUNG MAN Who Believed He Was Broken

A young man came to me convinced he was "broken." He described years of emptiness, failures, and isolation. His voice was flat, his posture defeated. He had seen other clinicians. He had tried medications. Nothing had helped for long.

The unwise approach would have been to diagnose quickly, intervene aggressively, and match symptoms to protocol. His presentation could have supported several diagnoses. A checklist would have found what it was looking for.

Instead, we slowed down. We explored the origins of his self-story. Where had he first learned that he was broken? Who had taught him that emptiness meant failure? What had happened in his early life that left him without a language for his own experience?

Over months, a different picture emerged. His "emptiness" was not a flaw in his character or his chemistry. It was the residue of emotional neglect—years of growing up in a home where his inner life was ignored, where his needs were treated as inconveniences, where he learned to disappear in order to survive.

As he developed language for his experience and compassion for himself, the emptiness receded. Not because it was treated, but because it was understood. He began to see that his suffering had a history, logic, and meaning. He was not broken. He had not failed.

Wisdom did what medication alone could not: it helped him reinterpret his life.

What Wisdom Offers That Knowledge Cannot

Knowledge categorizes. Skill intervenes. Protocols guide. Wisdom understands.

Knowledge can name a disorder. Skill can deliver treatment. Protocols can ensure consistency. But only wisdom can see the human being beneath the diagnostic language—the person who is more than their symptoms, more than their history, more than their worst days.

Wisdom recognizes that every patient arrives with a story already in progress, shaped by forces the clinician may never fully know. It approaches that story with curiosity rather than certainty, with humility rather than authority. It asks not only "What is wrong?" but "What has happened?" and "What does this person need in order to heal?"

And in doing so, wisdom opens a doorway to healing that no algorithm, checklist, or protocol can match. It restores to psychiatry what efficiency threatens to remove: the recognition that suffering is not merely a problem to be solved, but a human experience to be understood.

~

14

THE ART OF REINTERPRETATION

"We are not only the authors of our lives, but also the interpreters of what we have lived."
— Friedrich Nietzsche

Reinterpretation is not the rewriting of a patient's story— it is the uncovering of meanings that have long been buried beneath shame, fear, habit, or inherited narratives. People often live inside interpretations created in childhood, reinforced by family, culture, and experience. These interpretations feel like facts, not beliefs.

Most suffering arises not from events themselves, but from the meanings we learned to assign to them. Reinterpretation restores authorship to people who have lived inside inherited narratives. It invites patients to revise the stories that once protected them but now confine them.

Wisdom invites patients to examine the stories they have carried —the ones that shaped their identity without ever being questioned.

. . .

The Power of Giving Style to One's Character

Nietzsche wrote that humans must "give style" to their character —shape their experiences into a coherent narrative that reflects truth rather than fear. But many patients enter treatment with narratives shaped not by authenticity, but by survival.

A woman once told me, "I am unlovable."

She believed this not because it was true, but because it was the only interpretation that made sense in a childhood where affection was conditional. Love arrived unpredictably, withdrawn without warning, offered as reward, and withheld as punishment. The child made sense of this the only way she could: by deciding that the problem was her.

Through reinterpretation, she discovered that her belief was an adaptation, not an identity. The unlovability she had carried for decades was not a truth about her nature— it was a conclusion a child had drawn to survive an environment that offered no other explanation.

Reinterpretation does not distort reality. It liberates the patient from the interpretations they were forced to inherit.

Reinterpretation vs. Reframing

Reframing is cognitive. Reinterpretation is existential.

Reframing adjusts perspective. Reinterpretation reshapes identity.

Reframing asks: How else might you see this?

Reinterpretation asks: Who taught you to see yourself this way? What meaning did you give to this experience? What truth was present then that is not present now? What interpretation once protected you but now harms you?

The difference is depth. Reframing operates at the level of thought; reinterpretation operates at the level of self. A patient can reframe a single event and remain fundamentally unchanged. But when a patient reinterprets the narrative that has organized their identity, the ground shifts beneath them.

Reinterpretation shifts the foundation of the self.

THE TRUTH Beneath the Old Story

A man described himself as "weak" for feeling anxious in social situations. His father had mocked fear, teaching him that strength meant emotional silence. Any sign of vulnerability had been met with contempt. He learned early that safety required hiding.

Through reinterpretation, he began to understand that his anxiety was not weakness at all. It was hypervigilance—a survival response to years of unpredictability, a nervous system trained to scan for danger because danger had been real. His body had learned to protect him in the only way it knew how.

Once he reinterpreted his anxiety as evidence of adaptation rather than defect, something shifted. His shame loosened. His identity expanded. His capacity for growth increased. He was no longer a weak man fighting an irrational fear. He was a survivor whose body still carried the memory of what he had endured.

Reinterpretation revealed the truth beneath the old story.

WHEN INTERPRETATION BECOMES a Cage

Patients often cling to interpretations that harm them because those interpretations explain their suffering in a way that feels stable.

To relinquish an old interpretation can feel like losing a part of the self.

A woman who defined herself as "the caretaker" struggled to express need. Her self-worth and identity were bound to being indispensable. She had organized her entire life around the premise that her value lay in what she gave, never in what she required. To need something was to risk becoming dispensable.

Reinterpreting her role—not as duty but as choice—transformed her relationships and her sense of self. She began to see that caretaking had been a survival strategy, born in a family where her needs had been invisible. The role had protected her once. But it had also prevented her from experiencing the reciprocity that sustains connection.

Interpretations that once kept a person safe can become prisons later in life. Wisdom helps patients notice when meaning has become confinement.

THE CLINICIAN'S Role in Reinterpretation

The clinician's task is delicate. Reinterpretation must emerge from the patient's own exploration, not from the clinician's conviction.

This requires the clinician to avoid imposing meaning, to listen for the emotional truth beneath the patient's story, to honor the adaptive history behind the original interpretation, to guide gently toward alternative meanings, and to ensure that reinterpretation feels expansive rather than corrective.

Reinterpretation must never feel like erasure. It must feel like restoration.

The patient does not receive a new story. They reclaim the authorship of their old one. They come to discover that the meaning they had lived inside was not inevitable— it was constructed, under conditions they did not choose, by a younger self who was doing the best they could. And now, with more resources and more safety, they can construct again.

THE FREEDOM That Emerges

When patients reinterpret their past, they experience a profound internal shift. Shame softens. Agency expands. Self-compassion emerges. Identity becomes more spacious. Relationships become more authentic.

They begin to see themselves not as the product of their wounds, but as the interpreters of their experience. The past does not change —but its hold loosens. The story remains, but the patient is no longer trapped inside it.

Reinterpretation is the bridge between understanding and transformation. It is where wisdom becomes healing.

~

15

THE FUTURE OF
INSIGHT-BASED CARE

"The greatest discoveries are not new ideas, but new ways of seeing."
— Friedrich Nietzsche

Insight-based care is not nostalgic or antiquated. It is the future of psychiatry—especially as technology advances. Paradoxically, the more sophisticated our tools become, the more essential wisdom will be.

Psychiatry's future will depend not on new labels but on new perception. Insight—not information—is what transforms patients. The next evolution of mental health care will arise from the union of knowledge, context, and depth.

Technology expands what we can measure. Wisdom expands what we can understand.

WHERE TECHNOLOGY FALLS Short

Artificial intelligence can analyze patterns, predict risk, categorize symptoms, and detect linguistic cues. These capacities will continue to grow. Algorithms will become faster, more accurate, more comprehensive in their pattern recognition.

But technology cannot interpret emotion. It cannot sense contradiction or read silence. It cannot feel the weight of shame or discern cultural subtleties. It cannot understand identity conflicts or hold human grief with reverence.

Technology may assist, but it cannot replace the human capacity for emotional interpretation. Algorithms can see patterns. Only humans can see people.

Blending Data With Human Depth

The future of psychiatry lies in collaboration. Data identifies patterns. Clinicians interpret meaning. Patients bring emotional truth. Each contributes what the others cannot provide.

Technology will make diagnosis faster. Wisdom will make healing deeper.

A clinician who relies solely on data risks missing context—the story behind the symptom, the meaning beneath the behavior, the identity at stake in the diagnosis. A clinician who ignores data risks missing risk—the patterns that signal danger, the trends that indicate deterioration, the information that could protect a life.

The future belongs to those who can hold both: the precision of measurement and the depth of interpretation, the efficiency of technology and the patience of wisdom.

The Promise and Limits of Digital Tools

Digital tools hold genuine promise. They can improve early identification of distress, support patient self-awareness, reveal symptom trends over time, provide immediate feedback, and help track emotional patterns across weeks and months. For patients who struggle to articulate their experience in session, data gathered between appointments can open new avenues for understanding.

But no application can interpret why patterns matter.

A spike in irritability may reflect trauma activation, hormonal shift, interpersonal conflict, identity stress, cultural pressure, shame, or grief. The data shows the spike. Only the clinician—listening carefully, asking the right questions, holding the patient's history in mind—can discern what the spike means.

Applications provide information. Wisdom provides interpretation. Without a clinician who understands context, data becomes noise.

THE RISE of Personal Meaning in Treatment

As society becomes more psychologically aware, patients increasingly seek treatment that honors identity, culture, trauma, emotional nuance, and personal narrative. They arrive with questions that symptom checklists cannot answer. They want to know not only what is happening to them, but why it is happening and what it means.

Insight-based care will meet this need. It will move beyond symptom reduction toward meaning creation.

Patients no longer want to be told what they have. They want to understand why they hurt and who they can become. They seek clinicians who will engage with their full humanity—not merely their diagnoses—and who will help them construct narratives that make sense of their suffering and open pathways toward growth.

This is not a rejection of science. It is an expansion of what treatment is understood to offer.

· · ·

HUMBLER Psychiatry

The psychiatry of the future will require humility. It will mean acknowledging the limits of diagnostic systems, recognizing the variability of human expression, honoring personal meaning as much as biological explanation, treating protocols as guides rather than rules, and allowing patients to teach us how they suffer.

Insight-based care will shape a generation of clinicians who listen more deeply, interpret more wisely, diagnose more cautiously, and intervene more compassionately. These clinicians will understand that their expertise is not diminished by uncertainty—it is deepened by it. They will hold their knowledge lightly, remaining open to revision, attentive to what they do not yet understand.

Wisdom will become the discipline's defining skill—not its ornament.

The future of psychiatry is not a choice between science and humanity. It is the integration of both: rigorous in method, humble in posture, and always oriented toward the person who sits across the room, waiting to be understood.

∼

16

HOW WISDOM HEALS

"One must have chaos in oneself to give birth to a dancing star."
— Friedrich Nietzsche

W isdom heals not by offering answers, but by offering understanding. It creates the conditions in which truth becomes speakable and suffering becomes shareable. In this way, wisdom is not an intervention but an atmosphere—one in which clarity emerges naturally, safely, and at the pace the psyche can tolerate.

Healing is not the elimination of chaos but the transformation of it. Wisdom does not silence suffering—it helps suffering reorganize into meaning. The clinician's role is not to impose order, but to accompany the patient as truth becomes bearable.

Healing begins not with certainty, but with being understood.

Many patients improve the moment they feel understood—not fixed, not analyzed, but seen.

Wisdom sees the emotional architecture beneath symptoms: the fear beneath anger, the grief beneath irritability, the shame beneath silence, the longing beneath detachment. It perceives the logic of suffering even when that logic has never been articulated.

A patient once said to me, "I didn't know what I felt until you named it." The feeling had always been there- formless, pressing against the edges of awareness. But it had no shape, no permission to exist. Wisdom created space for it to emerge. The name was not an imposition. It was recognition.

To be seen is to become possible to oneself. When a patient is truly witnessed, something within them shifts. The isolation of suffering begins to dissolve. They discover that their inner world is not incomprehensible, not shameful, not too much. They discover that they can be known.

HEALING THROUGH INTERPRETATION

Interpretation is not theoretical. It is the act of making emotional life intelligible.

Through interpretation, patients learn to understand themselves, to recognize emotions they had hidden or disowned, to reclaim parts of the self they were taught to exile, to rewrite narratives they inherited but never chose, and to develop compassion for their own suffering.

Interpretation turns experience into meaning. Meaning turns symptoms into stories. Stories turn chaos into coherence.

A man who had always described himself as "angry" came to understand that his anger was grief—decades of unacknowledged loss compressed into the only emotion his family had permitted. A woman who called herself "too sensitive" came to see that her sensitivity was not a flaw but a capacity, shaped by early experiences that had required her to read emotional atmospheres for survival. In both cases, interpretation did not add something foreign. It uncovered something true.

Wisdom reorients the patient toward truth without shaming the defenses that once protected them. It honors the past while opening the future.

HEALING THROUGH RELATIONSHIP

The therapeutic relationship is not incidental. It is the medium of transformation.

When a patient feels safe enough to reveal what they have long hidden, the nervous system shifts. Shame loosens. Fear quiets. Grief surfaces. Identity expands. The body begins to learn what the mind may already suspect: that vulnerability does not always lead to harm.

Wisdom listens without fear of contradiction, without pressure for coherence, without the urgency to cure, without the haste that collapses complexity. It remains present through silence, through confusion, through the slow and often nonlinear movement toward truth.

The relationship becomes a rehearsal for a new way of being. Patients who have always hidden discover they can be visible. Patients who have always performed discover they can be real. Patients who have always protected others discover they can have needs of their own.

Through relationship, patients discover they can exist without hiding. And in that discovery, healing has already begun.

. . .

HEALING THROUGH WHOLENESS

Wisdom restores wholeness by gathering the patient's history, culture, identity, contradictions, symptoms, and emotional life into a single coherent narrative. It resists the fragmentation that diagnosis can impose, holding the patient as a complete person rather than a collection of problems.

People do not heal by erasing their past. They heal by integrating it.

Wholeness emerges when the clinician and patient together uncover what the patient truly feels, what the symptom protects, what the narrative hides, what the identity fears, and what meaning has been waiting to surface. This is not a checklist to be completed in a single session. It is the slow work of many conversations, many silences, many moments of recognition.

In this sense, wisdom is a form of dignifying. It restores complexity where shame created collapse. It returns to the patient the full range of their experience, including the parts they had learned to disown. Wholeness is not the absence of contradiction. It is the capacity to hold contradiction without being destroyed by it.

THE QUIET FORCE of Transformation

Psychiatry's deepest potential lies not only in reducing symptoms but in expanding the self.

Wisdom nurtures this expansion by illuminating the truths patients have carried without language. It helps them move from self-protection to self-understanding, from inherited meanings to chosen ones, from fragmentation to coherence. It does not rush this movement. It accompanies it.

Healing begins when people see themselves clearly—not with judgment, but with recognition. When a patient can look at their own history and understand why they became who they are, when they can feel compassion for the child who adapted in the only ways available, when they can distinguish between what was done to them and who they are—then healing has taken root.

Wisdom is the final diagnostic instrument. It sees what checklists miss and holds what protocols cannot contain. And in the quiet space it creates, understanding becomes changed.

~

VOLUME TWO

WISDOM IN PRESCRIBING

PART I

1

GENERAL PRINCIPLES OF PSYCHOPHARMACOLOGY

Introduction: Where Molecules Meet Meaning

P sychopharmacology lives at the intersection of two worlds: the intricate biological networks that shape mood, attention, and perception, and the lived experience of suffering, hope, and identity. To prescribe medication wisely is to move fluidly between these realms. It is never a purely technical act. It is a conversation about the nature of distress, the possibilities for change, and the meaning of relief.

Early in training, I learned that medication decisions begin with an exploration rather than a diagnosis. A mentor emphasized tracing a person's experience through a simple but powerful sequence: symptom, suffering, function, treatment. This lens shifted my focus from categorizing disorders to understanding how distress unfolds in life, how it constrains functioning, how it signals unmet needs, and what might restore balance. Over time, this way of thinking became foundational to my practice, reminding me that psychopharmacology is an art grounded in science and carried out in relationship.

THE PROMISE and the Paradox

Medications have transformed psychiatry. They can ease despair, soften anxiety, organize scattered thought, restore sleep, and modulate overwhelming emotion. And yet, their effect is characteristically partial. Across emotional and psychiatric disorders, medications typically reduce symptoms by fifty to seventy-five percent, and in more severe, chronic, or comorbid conditions, sometimes even less. But this partial relief can be life-altering. A patient who sleeps an additional hour, whose anxiety lessens enough to leave the house, or whose depression lifts just enough to participate in psychotherapy is not merely "somewhat improved"; they are newly able to engage in the world.

Psychiatric disorders reflect complex dysregulation of neural circuits, not simple "chemical imbalances." Medications influence these systems, but they do not fully normalize them. They reduce the intensity of symptoms enough to interrupt spirals, restore stability, and open space for psychological and relational healing.

One patient taught me this vividly. Medication restored a portion of her energy—perhaps half of what she once had—but that shift illuminated a grief she had long avoided. The medication opened a door; walking through it required emotional work, meaningful relationships, and time. Psychopharmacology requires us to hold this dual truth: medications matter deeply, and they are never the whole story.

THE ART of Relationship

Before a capsule is ever prescribed, the clinician must understand what relief means to the patient. For one person, medication is a bridge back to functioning; for another, a shield against overwhelming emotion; for another still, a sign that someone finally understands their pain.

This symbolic weight is not peripheral; it is central. A strong therapeutic alliance enhances adherence, amplifies placebo effects, and strengthens the patient's sense of agency. Sometimes, the effectiveness of a medication depends less on its mechanism of action than on the patient's experience of being seen and understood.

Psychopharmacology, in its essence, is a relational craft.

The Experience of Change

Although medications act through neurotransmitters, patients experience their effects in the realm of the self. A sedative may quiet the mind but dull enthusiasm. An antidepressant may restore motivation while raising questions about authenticity. A stimulant may sharpen focus while narrowing emotional spontaneity.

These shifts are not merely side effects—they are existential experiences. Patients describe them with nuance: "I feel more like myself." "I feel different, and I'm deciding if I like this version of me." "I feel clearer, but a little less passionate."

To guide patients well, clinicians must approach these changes with curiosity and humility. Medication modifies biology, but it also reshapes identity. Navigating this terrain thoughtfully is part of the work.

Preconceptions, Fears, and the Challenge of Adherence

Patients rarely approach medication from a neutral stance. Their beliefs are shaped by family, culture, past treatment experiences, and fears about losing autonomy or authenticity. Common concerns include fears that medication will change their personality, that they will no longer be themselves, that they will become dependent, that a higher dose signals something seriously wrong, or that they must know every possible side effect before taking anything.

These fears can overshadow even severe suffering. They arise from a desire to stay in control of one's own mind, a desire both understandable and worthy of respect.

Adherence adds complexity. When a patient says "Yes, I'm taking it," this may mean once every few days, only when symptoms worsen, only when they remember, or only when they believe they "really need it." Understanding patients' real medication patterns requires curiosity, not judgment.

Clinicians carry assumptions as well. For nearly a year, I avoided offering long acting injectables, convinced patients would reject them. When I finally offered them without hesitation or bias, most accepted immediately. One asked why I had waited so long. That moment revealed how clinician assumptions can delay relief.

Psychopharmacology is a landscape of interpretation—for both patient and clinician.

TRANSITION TO PRINCIPLES

With these relational and experiential foundations, we turn to the guiding principles of psychopharmacology. These principles are not algorithms, but frameworks grounded in clinical wisdom, humility, and attention to how symptoms, suffering, and functioning interact.

The Integrated Mental Health Screen (IMHS) offers a model of this thinking. It organizes symptoms across domains, understands severity as mild, moderate, or severe, assesses functioning directly, expects comorbidity rather than treating it as exceptional, and anchors medication decisions to severity combined with functional impairment rather than merely symptom presence. The IMHS integrates many underlying scales covering symptoms across different diagnostic and functional measurements in one place. It is available as an application at poe.com/mindcare1st.

This approach reinforces a central truth: medication decisions must reflect the whole person, not the diagnostic label alone.

I. Foundational Orientation

Medications as One Component of Comprehensive Care

Because medications typically provide partial—but meaningful —relief, their true value often lies in creating internal space for other forms of healing. Therapy becomes possible when anxiety abates enough for reflection. Behavioral interventions succeed when attention or irritability improves. Relational dynamics shift when emotional reactivity softens.

For children, this principle is especially clear. A medication that reduces aggression by even thirty to forty percent may allow a child to participate in preschool, benefit from early intervention, or access an Individualized Education Program—supports that promote developmental progress no medication alone can achieve.

Medication does not replace therapy, structure, safety, or environment. It supports them.

Respect for the Complexity of the Mind–Brain Relationship

Emotional and psychiatric disorders arise from dynamic interactions among biology, development, temperament, trauma, relationships, and environment. Medications influence brain circuits, but always within a larger context.

This complexity calls for humility.

. . .

II. Principles of Assessment Before Prescribing
Thorough Diagnostic Clarification

Effective prescribing begins with understanding what is happening—not just what it resembles diagnostically. Clinicians must differentiate psychiatric disorders from medical conditions, substance-induced symptoms, neurodevelopmental variations, and distress arising from context and circumstance.

The IMHS supports this process by illuminating patterns of symptoms, severity, and functional impact. Identifying target symptoms is essential.

Attention to Developmental Stage

Suffering expresses itself differently across ages. A preschooler shows distress through behavior. An adolescent through identity conflict or withdrawal. An older adult through slowed activity or somatic concerns.

Medication decisions must be tailored to the developmental meaning of symptoms, not simply their appearance.

Biopsychosocial Formulation

A sound formulation integrates biological vulnerabilities, psychological patterns, trauma history, relational systems, and sociocultural influences. This depth of understanding supports targeted, compassionate prescribing.

Risk–Benefit Evaluation

Medication becomes more essential when symptoms are moderate or severe, causing functional impairment, likely to recur, or compromising safety.

Untreated illness carries profound risks, often greater than those of medication.

. . .

III. Principles of Initiating Medication

Start Low, Go Slow—But Go

Titration should be thoughtful, yet clinicians should not hesitate to reach therapeutic doses. Under-treatment prolongs suffering unnecessarily.

Clear, Shared Treatment Goals

A realistic therapeutic expectation is significant reduction in suffering, not eradication of symptoms. Aiming for thirty to seventy percent improvement aligns with what medications typically provide and prevents discouragement when symptoms persist.

The IMHS framework—linking symptoms to functional disruption—helps clarify these goals.

Informed Consent and Collaborative Decision-Making

Patients deserve clear, accessible explanations of expected benefits, potential side effects, timelines, and alternatives. Collaboration strengthens trust and autonomy.

Respect for Patient Values and Autonomy

Medication decisions must honor the patient's beliefs, culture, fears, and hopes. Respect is itself therapeutic.

IV. Principles of Monitoring and Adjustment

Systematic Follow-Up

Close monitoring allows clinicians to evaluate symptoms, side effects, functioning, and adherence. Structure and conversation complement one another.

Therapeutic Alliance as a Clinical Tool

Medication works best within trust. Ongoing dialogue allows patients to express ambivalence and participate actively in their care.

Titration and Optimization

Dose adjustments should reflect therapeutic response, tolerability, and evolving understanding. Premature switching may obscure unrealized benefit.

Managing Side Effects

Side effects must be addressed promptly and proportionally. When a patient reports a troubling effect, the clinician's response— whether adjusting the dose, changing the timing, adding a counter-measure, or switching medications—communicates that the patient's experience matters. Dismissing side effects erodes trust; attending to them strengthens the alliance and improves adherence.

CLOSING **Reflection**

The principles outlined in this chapter are not rules to be followed mechanically. They are orientations— ways of thinking that keep the patient at the center of psychopharmacological care. Medications are powerful tools, but their power is realized only within a framework of understanding, relationship, and respect for the complexity of human suffering.

The chapters that follow will apply these principles to specific conditions and clinical situations. But the foundation remains constant: psychopharmacology is most effective when it is most human.

∽

PART II

2

PSYCHOPHARMACOLOGY IN PRESCHOOLERS

I. Thematic Reflection: When Behavior Speaks for the Self

In early childhood, emotion and action are inseparable. A preschooler cannot say, "I am overwhelmed" or "I am frightened by the force of my own feelings." Instead, distress becomes motion—throwing, biting, hitting, collapsing, fleeing. Their internal world is expressed through the body, and their suffering is revealed in behaviors that adults may experience as chaotic or alarming.

For the clinician, the work is not simply to describe symptoms but to interpret the meaning behind these movements: fear, frustration, the developmental vulnerability. Medication, when considered, enters this deeply human landscape—one defined as much by the child's unspoken struggle as by the parents' hopes, doubts, and fears.

II. Developmental Overview: The Preschool Brain Under Strain

Preschool years are marked by rapid neurodevelopment. Emotional intensity is high; regulation capacity is limited; behavior is communication. The nervous system is highly plastic but highly vulnerable. When persistent dysregulation overwhelms the child's limited capacity to cope, development can stall.

At this age, emotional regulation remains primitive and impulse control is minimal. Attachment and environment play central roles in shaping the child's experience. Behavior serves as the primary language of distress. Medication is never the starting point—but at times, suffering and safety demand that it becomes part of the treatment plan.

III. Clinical Vignette: When Safety Becomes the Threshold

Jacob was four years old and moved through the world like a storm. In frustration, he lunged, bit, hit, or shoved with striking force. His teachers rearranged the classroom to minimize risk. His parents alternated between fear and exhaustion. Jacob often cried afterward, frightened by his own intensity.

The decision to use medication was agonizing for his parents. They feared judgment and felt a sense of defeat, "Shouldn't we be able to help him without medication?" Their ambivalence persisted even after consenting to treatment.

What ultimately shifted the conversation was the recognition that Jacob's safety—and the safety of others—was at risk. Once medication was introduced, the change was not dramatic but meaningful. His aggression softened. He paused before striking. He remained in the classroom long enough to participate in early intervention and therapeutic activities. Relief spread through the ecosystem of his life.

Medication did not change who Jacob was; it lowered the emotional intensity enough for development to re-engage.

. . .

IV. Integrating Clinical Insight: The Meaning of Medication in Early Childhood

Choosing medication for a preschooler is emotionally complex. Parents commonly experience fear, shame, doubt, and a sense of failure. They may worry about long-term consequences or whether their child is being "drugged."

A central truth helps guide these decisions: when suffering and risk exceed the child's developmental capacity to cope, medication may be a compassionate, necessary, and stabilizing intervention.

Medication does not replace developmental work. It creates space for it.

V. Understanding Suffering in Preschoolers

Suffering in early childhood is often misinterpreted as misbehavior. Yet beneath the surface of explosive tantrums, hitting, biting, or bolting is almost always distress. These behaviors reflect emotional overload beyond the child's regulatory capacity.

Preschool suffering commonly appears through aggression, explosive tantrums, self-injury, severe irritability, sleep disruption, sensory overstimulation, and clinginess or fearfulness. A child is not "misbehaving"; a child is flooded.

VI. Assessment Framework: Applying IMHS Logic to Early Childhood

The Integrated Mental Health Screen reasoning process can be adapted to preschoolers through five interconnected dimensions.

The first dimension is symptoms. The clinician describes observable behaviors—their frequency, intensity, and triggers. The second dimension is suffering. The clinician assesses emotional distress even when the child cannot verbalize it, reading the child's experience through behavior, affect, and physiological signs. The third dimension is functioning. Key domains include safety, play, learning, relationships, and the ability to remain in the classroom. The fourth dimension is severity, which is determined by frequency, intensity, predictability, recovery time, and risk. The fifth dimension is comorbidity. Common contributors include trauma, sensory dysregulation, developmental delays, mood dysregulation, and anxiety.

Medication decisions emerge from understanding the whole pattern—not isolated behaviors.

VII. When Medication Becomes Necessary

Medication is reserved for circumstances where suffering and risk are substantial.

The first circumstance is severe aggression compromising safety. This includes biting, hitting, throwing objects, choking, or attacking caregivers. These behaviors require swift, compassionate intervention. The second circumstance is severe dysregulation blocking participation in school or therapy. If a child cannot remain in the classroom or engage in early intervention, developmental opportunities are lost. The third circumstance is persistent, intense distress despite robust environmental and therapeutic support. When a child continues to struggle despite multiple interventions, medication becomes a reasonable next step.

Parents typically agree only when the necessity becomes undeniable.

.   .   .

VIII. Principles of Prescribing in Preschoolers

Prescribing for young children requires exceptional care.

The first principle is to start low, go slow—but go. Titration should be thoughtful and steady, moving toward therapeutic benefit without unnecessary delay. The second principle is to treat target symptoms rather than diagnostic labels. Aggression, irritability, hyperarousal, and sleep disruption are the meaningful targets. The third principle is to use the smallest number of medications possible; polypharmacy is rarely justified at this age. The fourth principle is to combine medication with intensive environmental supports. Medication alone is insufficient; it opens the door for real learning. The fifth principle is to educate parents thoroughly. Understanding realistic expectations prevents disappointment and improves adherence. The sixth principle is to monitor frequently. Preschoolers change rapidly and require close observation.

Rapid Metabolism and Dosing Principles in Young Children

Young children metabolize medications rapidly—often faster than adults relative to body weight. Parents are frequently surprised to learn that their preschooler may require a higher milligram-per-kilogram dose than intuition suggests. This is not because they are receiving "more" in a concerning sense, but because their bodies process medication quickly.

A calm, clear explanation helps parents understand this developmental reality. Doses must be matched to the child's rate of metabolism, not to adult assumptions about weight-based proportionality.

The guiding therapeutic rule remains use the lowest dose that produces the maximum benefit with the least—or no—side effects.

This approach reassures families while supporting thoughtful, effective titration.

IX. Neurobiological Rationale: Medication as a Support for Plasticity

During preschool years, neural circuits for regulation, attention, and emotional learning are actively forming. When dysregulation overwhelms the system, development slows. Medication can reduce emotional overload and create conditions in which neuroplasticity thrives.

Medication does not create skills, but it creates access to the environments and experiences that build those skills.

X. GENETIC TESTING: Guiding Treatment When Response Is Limited

When a young child does not respond as expected to medication —or experiences side effects at unusually low doses—genetic testing can offer valuable insight. Pharmacogenomic testing helps clarify how a child metabolizes medications and whether certain genetic markers suggest a more or less favorable response.

Genetic testing is especially useful in several circumstances: when multiple medication trials have produced limited or inconsistent benefit, when side effects appear rapidly or unexpectedly, when there is a mismatch between dose and response, or when clinicians are deciding between several plausible medication options.

While not a standalone decision-making tool, pharmacogenomic information can reduce uncertainty, prevent unnecessary trial-and-error, and support safer, more individualized prescribing.

The guiding principle remains unchanged: choose the medication that offers maximum benefit with minimal burden, using genetic data as one more piece of a thoughtful, comprehensive approach.

XI. Medication Classes and Clinical Considerations

Several medication classes are used in preschool psychopharmacology, each with specific indications and considerations.

Alpha-agonists such as guanfacine and clonidine are helpful for aggression, irritability, hyperarousal, and sleep issues. These medications reduce sympathetic nervous system activation and can soften the intensity of emotional storms without causing significant sedation at appropriate doses.

Stimulants are useful for ADHD-like symptoms when attention difficulties, hyperactivity, and impulsivity are prominent features of the clinical picture. Careful diagnosis is essential, as many preschool behaviors that resemble ADHD reflect developmental immaturity, anxiety, or trauma rather than the disorder itself.

Atypical antipsychotics are reserved for severe aggression or self-injury that has not responded to other interventions. These medications require careful monitoring for metabolic effects, weight gain, and movement abnormalities.

SSRIs are used cautiously for severe anxiety or trauma-related symptoms. When a preschooler's distress is rooted in fear, separation anxiety, or traumatic experience, and when that distress significantly impairs functioning despite environmental and therapeutic intervention, SSRIs may provide meaningful relief.

XII. Environment, Therapy, and School Supports

Medication lowers emotional intensity; environment builds capacity. Preschoolers benefit from early intervention services, occupational and speech therapy, parent–child therapy, structured routines, consistent behavioral strategies, sensory supports, and Individualized Education Programs when necessary.

Medication makes participation possible; the environment shapes the outcome.

XIII. Parent–Clinician Relationship: Navigating Ambivalence

Parents often feel fear, shame, or guilt when medication becomes part of their child's treatment. The clinician's task is to meet these feelings with empathy and clarity.

A helpful frame is: "You are not failing your child. You are reducing their suffering so they can grow."

This reframing does not dismiss parental concerns but honors them while offering a different perspective. The decision to use medication can be an act of love rather than a sign of defeat. Partnership strengthens adherence and deepens trust. When parents feel heard and respected, they become active collaborators in their child's care rather than reluctant participants.

XIV. Additional Vignette: A Small Shift, A Big Change

Maya, age three, had daily meltdowns so severe she vomited. Her parents had tried everything they could think of—consistent routines, sensory strategies, reduced demands—but her distress continued unabated. After starting a low-dose alpha-agonist, her distress decreased by nearly half. She could remain in her classroom. She made eye contact again. A forty to fifty percent improvement transformed her developmental trajectory.

Maya's story illustrates a recurring theme in preschool psychopharmacology: partial improvement is often profound improvement. When a child moves from constant crisis to manageable difficulty, the entire ecosystem of their life shifts. Parents regain hope. Teachers find strategies which work. Therapists gain traction. The child begins to learn.

XV. Closing Reflection: Opening Space for Development

Preschool psychopharmacology is not about eliminating symptoms—it is about lowering distress to a level where growth becomes possible. Even partial improvement can alter a child's trajectory and restore safety, connection, and learning.

The preschool years are a window of extraordinary plasticity. What happens during this period shapes the architecture of the developing brain. When a child is trapped in cycles of dysregulation, that window narrows. Medication, used thoughtfully and in combination with environmental and therapeutic supports, can keep the window open.

Medication opens the door. Development walks through it.

PSYCHOPHARMACOLOGY IN SCHOOL-AGE CHILDREN (AGES 6–11)

I. Thematic Reflection: The Burden of Expectation

B y the time a child enters school, the world begins to expect things of them. Sit still. Pay attention. Follow the rules. Share. Wait your turn. Use your words. Control yourself. Be patient. Learn on schedule. Behave predictably.

These expectations create a profound shift in the child's internal landscape. A child who struggled quietly at home may suddenly be overwhelmed in the classroom. A child who was merely "active" in preschool may now be seen as "disruptive." Meanwhile, the child becomes increasingly aware of peers, rules, and social judgment.

At this stage, suffering becomes more self-aware. The child begins to ask questions that reveal a dawning and painful consciousness: "Why can't I do what the other kids do?" "Why am I always in trouble?" "Why can't I control it?"

Psychopharmacology in this age group is not only about reducing symptoms—it is about protecting identity, preserving confidence, and mitigating the shame that can take root when a child feels chronically inadequate.

II. Developmental Overview: The Expanding Mind of the School-Age Child

Between ages six and eleven, children's cognitive, emotional, and social capacities expand dramatically. Language becomes more precise, allowing children to articulate experiences that previously could only be expressed through behavior. Self-observation increases, and with it comes a new capacity for both insight and self-criticism. Peer comparison intensifies as children measure themselves against classmates and friends. School demands escalate year by year, requiring sustained attention, behavioral regulation, and cognitive flexibility. Moral awareness develops, bringing with it the capacity for guilt, shame, and a sense of justice.

This means psychological suffering becomes both felt more deeply and understood more consciously. Children in this age group are not simply behaving—they are interpreting themselves. A child who struggles is no longer merely struggling; they are forming conclusions about who they are.

III. Clinical Vignette: Understanding the Child Behind the Chaos

Ethan, age eight, was bright and curious, but in school his intensity became a crisis. He blurted answers, wandered the room, bumped into peers, forgot assignments, and erupted in frustration. By midyear, he spent more time in the hallway than in class.

At home, his parents were heartbroken. They had tried every

parenting strategy available. Ethan himself often asked, "Why am I the kid who gets in trouble?"

When medication was discussed, his parents were fearful—shaped by cultural judgment, personal experiences, and societal stigma. Ethan simply asked, "Will it help me not get in trouble so much?"

Within weeks of treatment, Ethan shared a reflection that captures the meaning of medication for this age group: "I can catch myself now. Before, it was like my body moved before I thought."

Medication did not change Ethan's personality— it gave him access to regulation, control, and dignity.

IV. The Expanding Emotional Landscape: Self-Image and Pressure

School-age children navigate multiple systems simultaneously. They must meet family expectations while also adapting to classroom rules. They receive teacher evaluations that shape their sense of academic competence. They internalize peer norms that define social belonging. They face early academic pressures that will only intensify as they progress through school.

Failure to meet expectations now affects self-worth in ways that were not possible during preschool years. Children may experience guilt when they disappoint adults, shame when they fall short of their own expectations, embarrassment when peers witness their struggles, or fear of being labeled "the bad kid."

Medication decisions must consider the identity-level consequences of untreated suffering. A child whose symptoms remain unaddressed is not simply continuing to struggle behaviorally—they are forming a narrative about themselves that may persist long after the symptoms themselves would have been treatable.

. . .

V. Complex Presentations: ADHD, Anxiety, Mood, and Bipolarity

Symptoms expand in complexity during middle childhood, and clinical presentations often involve multiple overlapping conditions.

Attention-deficit/hyperactivity disorder becomes more visible as demands on attention and behavior increase. A child who managed adequately in the more flexible environment of early childhood may decompensate when faced with the structured expectations of elementary school. The core features of inattention, hyperactivity, and impulsivity become increasingly reducing functioning as academic and social demands intensify.

Anxiety may present itself in ways that mimic other conditions. An anxious child may appear inattentive because worry consumes their mental bandwidth. They may seem irritable because chronic anxiety depletes their regulatory resources. They may complain of stomachaches or headaches because their distress is expressed somatically. Recognizing anxiety beneath surface presentations prevents misdiagnosis and inappropriate treatment.

Aggression frequently masks underlying anxiety or mood dysregulation. A child who fights or threatens may be experiencing internal states they cannot name or manage. The behavioral surface does not always reveal the emotional depth beneath it. Careful assessment explores what drives aggression rather than simply targeting its expression.

Mood swings are common during middle childhood and are often misunderstood without developmental context. Children's emotional lives are naturally more variable than adults. However, when mood instability exceeds developmental norms—when it impairs functioning, disrupts relationships, or causes significant distress—clinical attention is warranted.

Bipolar disorder can emerge during middle childhood and may

mimic ADHD or coexist with it. Indicators that raise concern for bipolarity include a decreased need for sleep without corresponding fatigue, grandiosity or inflated self-regard that exceeds typical childhood confidence, episodic intensity that differs qualitatively from the child's baseline, and dramatic mood shifts that cannot be explained by context alone. Careful assessment is crucial to avoid misdiagnosis and inappropriate stimulant escalation, which can destabilize mood in children with bipolar vulnerability.

VI. Assessment Using IMHS Logic in Middle Childhood

The Integrated Mental Health Screen reasoning process applies to school-age children with adaptations that reflect their developmental capacities.

The first dimension is symptoms. The clinician describes behavior across settings, recognizing that school-age children may present differently at home, in school, and with peers. Cross-setting information is essential for accurate diagnosis.

The second dimension is suffering. Unlike preschoolers, school-age children can often articulate their distress when asked directly. Questions like "How does it feel when you can't focus?" or "What is it like when you get in trouble?" can yield rich clinical information. The child's own words carry diagnostic weight.

The third dimension is functioning. Key domains include school performance, peer relationships, and family dynamics. The clinician assesses whether the child is learning, whether they have friends, whether home life is stable or strained by the child's symptoms.

The fourth dimension is severity. Severity is determined by impact on self-esteem, social standing, consistency of impairment, and safety concerns. A child who is failing academically, losing friends, and beginning to see themselves as defective is experiencing severe impairment regardless of how their symptoms might appear on a checklist.

The fifth dimension is comorbidity. In school-age children, comorbidity is the norm rather than the exception. Most children who present for psychiatric evaluation have more than one condition, and treatment planning must address the full clinical picture.

VII. When Medication Becomes Necessary

Medication may be appropriate when suffering significantly impairs development, when symptoms lead to repeated failure in academic or social domains, when self-esteem is compromised by chronic difficulties, when aggression threatens safety, when learning becomes impossible despite robust support, or when mood instability disrupts functioning across settings.

The decision to use medication is not about improving performance or making a child more convenient for adults. It is about reducing suffering and protecting identity. A child who cannot access their own potential because of untreatable symptoms deserves consideration of all available interventions, including medication.

VIII. The Child's Voice in Medication Decisions

Unlike preschoolers, school-age children can participate meaningfully in treatment decisions. They can express preferences about whether they want to try medication. They can ask informed questions about what medication will do and what side effects might occur. They can describe internal states with increasing precision, providing feedback that guides titration. They can identify benefits and side effects that adults might miss.

Many children recognize their own improvement quickly and

become advocates for their treatment. Some remind clinicians at follow-up visits: "Don't forget my refill. It helps me at school." This stands in contrast to the fears often carried by adults, who bear the weight of stigma, judgment, and their own histories with mental health treatment.

Including the child's voice in medication decisions respects their developing autonomy and improves treatment engagement. A child who understands why they are taking medication and who experiences its benefits firsthand becomes a partner in their own care.

IX. Genetic Testing: Guiding Treatment When Response Is Limited

When a school-age child does not respond as expected to medication—or experiences side effects at unusually low doses—genetic testing can offer valuable insight. Pharmacogenomic testing helps clarify how a child metabolizes medications and whether certain genetic markers suggest a more or less favorable response.

Genetic testing is especially useful when multiple medication trials have produced limited or inconsistent benefit, when side effects appear rapidly or unexpectedly, when there is a mismatch between dose and response, or when clinicians are deciding between several plausible medication options.

While not a standalone decision-making tool, pharmacogenomic information can reduce uncertainty, prevent unnecessary trial-and-error, and support safer, more individualized prescribing.

The guiding principle remains unchanged: choose the medication that offers maximum benefit with minimal burden, using genetic data as one more piece of a thoughtful, comprehensive approach.

. . .

X. Medication Principles in School-Age Children

Several principles guide use of medication in this age group.

The first principle is to start low, go slow, and adjust with clarity. Titration should be methodical, with clear communication to families about what to expect and when to report back.

The second principle is to target symptoms rather than diagnostic labels. The goal is reduction of suffering and improvement in functioning, not the treatment of an abstract category.

The third principle involves thoughtful selection among medication classes. Stimulants remain first-line treatment for ADHD and impulsivity when the diagnosis is clear. Alpha-agonists such as guanfacine and clonidine address irritability, aggression, and hyperarousal, and may be used alone or in combination with stimulants. SSRIs are effective for anxiety and obsessive-compulsive symptoms, which are common in this age group. Mood stabilizers and atypical antipsychotics are reserved for bipolar presentations or severe aggression that have not responded to other interventions.

The fourth principle is that partial improvement is meaningful. A forty to sixty percent reduction in symptoms can transform school life, restore peer relationships, and protect self-esteem. Clinicians should not pursue perfection at the cost of tolerability.

The fifth principle is to monitor side effects closely. Appetite suppression, sleep disruption, irritability, and behavioral activation all require attention. School-age children can often report these experiences themselves, and their feedback should be actively solicited.

XI. Comprehensive Treatment: Medication as One Component

Medication works best when integrated with a comprehensive treatment approach. Behavioral therapy provides structure and reinforcement for adaptive behaviors. Cognitive-behavioral therapy addresses anxiety, mood symptoms, and maladaptive thought patterns. Family therapy strengthens the home environment and improves parent-child relationships. Structured routines reduce unpredictability and support regulation. Sleep hygiene addresses a foundation of mental health that is often disrupted in struggling children. Individualized Education Programs or 504 accommodations ensure that school expectations are matched to the child's capacities. Social skills interventions address peer difficulties that may persist even after other symptoms improve. Teacher collaboration ensures consistency between home and school approaches.

Medication enables participation in these interventions; it does not replace them. A child who cannot sit still long enough to engage in therapy, who cannot regulate enough to benefit from behavioral strategies, or who cannot focus enough to learn from instruction may need medication to access the treatments that will ultimately build lasting skills.

XII. Closing Reflection: Protecting the Developing Self

The school-age years revolve around learning how to belong. Children are discovering where they fit—in their families, in their classrooms, among their peers, in the larger world. When suffering overwhelms a child during this period, the risk extends far beyond academic difficulties. The deeper danger is the internalization of shame: "I can't do anything right."

Psychopharmacology in this age group is not simply symptom management—it is protection of the developing self. It restores hope when a child has begun to despair. It rebuilds competence when a child has begun to doubt their abilities. It repairs connection when a child has begun to withdraw from relationships. It allows children to experience themselves not as problems to be managed, but as capable beings navigating a complex world.

Medication opens space for growth. Development fills it with possibility.

4

PSYCHOPHARMACOLOGY
IN ADOLESCENCE

Adolescence is a developmental threshold marked by rapid neurobiological change, expanding social complexity, and the emergence of a more differentiated sense of self. In psychopharmacology, this period presents a unique convergence of opportunity and vulnerability. Medications can be powerfully effective in alleviating suffering, restoring function, and enabling developmental momentum—but they can also disrupt emerging identity, strain family relationships, or create unintended consequences if used without careful attention to context.

For clinicians, this age group is both challenging and deeply fascinating. Adolescents speak a language of their own—part literal, part symbolic—and often communicate more through tone, posture, or silence than through tidy narratives. Working with them requires attunement to subtlety, flexibility in approach, and sensitivity to their rapidly shifting states of mind.

Wisdom in prescribing for adolescents requires more than knowledge of pharmacodynamics. It calls for an appreciation of their interior world, the multiple pressures acting upon them, and the developmental tasks they are simultaneously attempting to negotiate.

I. DEVELOPMENTAL CONSIDERATIONS: The Brain in Transition

The adolescent brain is in the midst of synaptic pruning and myelination, with frontal-striatal circuits still developing into the mid-twenties. Emotional reactivity can outpace executive control. These dynamics complicate both clinical presentation and medication response.

But adolescence is also a time of internal conflict. The push toward autonomy collides with dependency needs. Identity formation intersects with insecurity. Impulse-driven reward seeking must somehow coexist with emerging long-term planning. Many symptoms—irritability, impulsiveness, mood lability—exist at the intersection of neurobiology and developmental demands.

Clinically, this means that what looks like pathology may partially reflect the struggle to reconcile internal drives with external expectations. The clinician must hold open the question of whether a given presentation represents disorder, development, or some admixture of both.

II. Diagnosis in Adolescence: A Meeting of Two Stories

Diagnosing adolescents is uniquely challenging because the parent's account and the adolescent's account frequently differ—not only in details but in priorities. Parents often see impact on functioning: academic performance, household responsibilities, emotional volatility. Adolescents describe internal states: feeling overwhelmed, misunderstood, pressured, or numb.

Both perspectives are true, each shaped by different vantage points. The clinician becomes the interpreter of these parallel narratives, listening for patterns, tensions, and the deeper story beneath the surface.

Adolescents also live complex, multilayered lives. They navigate academic pressure while simultaneously grappling with identity questions. They negotiate peer hierarchies while managing family conflict. They exist within social media landscapes that amplify comparison, judgment, and performance anxiety. Development itself is a demanding full-time job. Symptoms often reflect not only internal vulnerability but also the strain of reconciling these intersecting demands.

A wise diagnostic stance recognizes that understanding emerges through relationship, curiosity, and time—not through checklist-style questioning alone. The clinician who rushes to diagnosis may miss the developmental context that gives symptoms their meaning.

III. The Meaning of Medication in Adolescence

Medication carries psychological weight during this developmental period that it may not carry at other ages. Adolescents may wonder whether taking medication means they are no longer truly themselves, whether needing medication means weakness, or whether others will judge them for requiring pharmaceutical support. These questions are not incidental; they touch the core developmental tasks of identity formation and social belonging.

Meanwhile, parents may struggle with their own complex feelings: fear about their child's suffering, hope that medication will help, guilt about whether they contributed to the problem, and urgency to see improvement before consequences accumulate.

Medication thus becomes more than a treatment—it becomes a symbol interacting with identity, autonomy, and belonging. Understanding that symbolic role helps clinicians frame medication in a way that reduces shame and increases collaboration. A clinician who ignores the meaning of medication prescribes into a vacuum; one who addresses it directly creates space for genuine engagement.

IV. Principles of Wise Prescribing for Adolescents

Several principles guide effective psychopharmacology during this developmental period.

Building Rapport by Honoring Adolescent Priorities

Adolescents are far more willing to engage when they feel the clinician is attending to what they want—not only what parents and schools demand. A clinician might begin with something like: "Let's work on the things that matter to you first. At the same time, we'll try to help you meet the expectations that feel unavoidable."

This reframing often generates immediate relief and trust. Adolescents rarely object to working on adult priorities as long as their own goals are also treated as legitimate. The clinician who begins with parental concerns and adds adolescent concerns as an afterthought has already compromised the alliance.

Navigating the Triangle

Medication decisions in adolescence occur within a triad of competing expectations involving the adolescent, parents, and often the school. Success frequently depends on helping adolescents achieve their own aims while simultaneously supporting parents and schools in maintaining safety and functioning. This requires diplomatic skill, clear communication, and sometimes the willingness to hold tension without premature resolution.

Addressing Adherence by Understanding Its Meaning

Adherence is particularly challenging in adolescence—not simply because of forgetfulness, but because taking medication touches autonomy, identity, and stigma. Non-adherence often carries meaning that deserves exploration rather than correction. An adolescent who stops taking medication may be asserting control over their own body. They may be avoiding feeling differently from peers. They may remain unconvinced that medication actually helps. They may be enacting opposition to parents through the medication relationship.

Exploring these meanings strengthens adherence far more than reminders or lectures. The clinician who asks, "What would it mean to you to take this medication every day?" learns more than one who simply reviews the prescription instructions.

Providing Information in Their Language

Adolescents respond best to explanations that are concrete, non-patronizing, and linked to their immediate goals. Abstract discussions of neurotransmitters matter less than clear statements about how medication might affect sleep, focus, mood, relationships, or performance. Clinical wisdom lies in speaking with adolescents, not at them—treating them as collaborators in their own care rather than passive recipients of adult decisions.

V. The Landscape of Risk: Substance Use and Peer Influence

Peer culture during adolescence can amplify impulsivity and experimentation. This reality significantly increases the risk of substance use and misuse, including exposure to vaping, cannabis, and alcohol. Risk-taking behaviors become more common when reinforced by peer approval. Medication diversion—sharing or selling prescribed medications—becomes a real concern, particularly with controlled substances. Self-harm behaviors can spread through contagion effects in certain peer or online groups.

These behaviors interact with medication in complex ways.

Substance use may blunt medication effectiveness or potentiate dangerous side effects. It may mask underlying psychiatric vulnerability, making accurate diagnosis more difficult. It may create medical emergencies when substances interact with prescribed medications.

Understanding peer dynamics is therefore not optional; it is central to safe prescribing. The clinician must inquire about substance use without judgment, assess diversion risk honestly, and factor peer context into treatment planning. An adolescent's social environment is not background information—it is part of the clinical picture.

VI. The Therapeutic Alliance as Container and Compass

Adolescents engage when they feel seen. Rapport is rarely built through technique alone—it emerges when clinicians show authenticity, respect, and attunement to the adolescent's experience.

Several guiding principles support the alliance. The clinician should ask the adolescent first, allowing them to lead the narrative before turning to parents for additional information. The clinician should validate the adolescent's dilemmas even when limits must be set—acknowledging the difficulty of a situation does not mean endorsing every choice. The clinician should collaborate on treatment decisions wherever possible, recognizing that adolescents who participate in decisions are more likely to follow through on them. The clinician should maintain consistent boundaries that offer safety without rigidity, providing structure that reduce anxiety rather than provoking rebellion.

When adolescents feel that treatment aligns with their emerging sense of self, they participate more openly, and medication becomes part of a larger developmental journey rather than an imposed solution. The alliance is not merely a nice addition to pharmacology—it is the context within which pharmacology becomes meaningful.

VII. Medication as One Thread in a Larger Tapestry

Medication may reduce suffering, but it cannot complete the developmental tasks of adolescence. It cannot resolve peer conflict or soothe existential uncertainty. It cannot replace needed guidance, connection, or the slow accumulation of life experience. Its role is to create enough internal stability so that adolescents can continue the work of becoming themselves.

In that sense, psychopharmacology must be practiced with humility. It is not the center of treatment—it is a support that enables the unfolding of the adolescent's growth. The clinician who over-promises medication's effects sets up disappointment; the one who positions medication accurately—as helpful but partial—maintains credibility and realistic expectations.

Comprehensive treatment during adolescence typically includes psychotherapy in various forms, family work to address relational patterns, school accommodations when needed, attention to sleep and physical health, and support for the adolescent's own efforts at self-understanding. Medication supports these efforts; it does not substitute for them.

VIII. Discontinuation: Knowing When to Consider It

Discontinuation should be thoughtful, gradual, and jointly planned. Not every adolescent who begins medication will need it indefinitely, and many will appropriately question whether they still require pharmacological support as they mature.

Candidates for tapering include adolescents who have sustained improvement for several months, who have engaged in psychotherapy and developed coping skills, who are entering a new developmental phase such as transitioning to college, or who express a desire to understand themselves without medication. These motivations deserve respect rather than reflexive discouragement.

A careful taper respects both neurobiological realities and the adolescent's psychological needs. Abrupt discontinuation risks destabilization: gradual reduction allows monitoring of emerging symptoms. The process itself can become an opportunity for growth and reflection, as the adolescent learns to observe their own internal states and recognize early warning signs.

When discontinuation reveals the return of significant symptoms, this information is valuable rather than discouraging. It clarifies the ongoing role of medication and may increase the adolescent's appreciation of its benefits.

IX. Closing Reflection

Practicing psychopharmacology with wisdom during adolescence is to honor the adolescent's unfolding identity, the family's hopes and fears, and the neurodevelopmental context in which symptoms arise. Medication can be a powerful ally, reducing suffering and enabling developmental progress. Yet it must be used with sensitivity, humility, and a commitment to partnership.

The goal is not merely symptom control but the support of an adolescent's journey toward resilience, self-understanding, and a sense of agency. In this way, psychopharmacology becomes not only a medical intervention but an instrument of healing within a broader developmental story.

5

MOOD DISORDERS IN CHILDHOOD AND ADOLESCENCE

SEEING THE UNSEEN, HEARING THE UNSAID

T his chapter addresses one of the most consequential gaps in psychiatric practice: the underrecognition of Mood Disorders in children and adolescents. It follows naturally from Chapter 4's examination of psychiatric treatment across the lifespan, but the subject demands dedicated attention. The stakes are too high, the patterns of missed diagnosis too entrenched, and the consequences of failure too lasting to treat this topic as a subsection of broader developmental material.

Mood Disorders in youth occupy a peculiar position in psychiatry. The evidence for their existence is robust. The suffering they cause is immense. The treatments available are often effective. Yet diagnosis remains delayed, sometimes by years, sometimes by decades. Children cycle through labels—ADHD, oppositional defiant disorder, anxiety, behavioral problems, difficult temperament—before anyone names what is actually happening. Adolescents receive antidepressants that destabilize them, conclude that treatment is harmful, and withdraw from care. Families exhaust themselves seeking help that does not come.

This chapter exists because these failures are not inevitable. Mood Disorders in youth can be recognized if clinicians know what to look for. They can be distinguished from conditions they resemble if the right questions are asked. They can be treated effectively if treatment is appropriate to the actual diagnosis. And young lives can be transformed when these things happen.

The chapter draws on clinical experience across generations, the patterns that repeat in families, the presentations that evolve from preverbal childhood through adolescence, the treatment relationships that span years. It offers vignettes not as curiosities but as illustrations of principles that apply broadly. It provides diagnostic guidance not as algorithm but as orientation to a complex clinical landscape.

Above all, it argues for a stance: that clinicians working with children and adolescents must be willing to see what is often unseen and hear what is frequently unsaid. Mood Disorders hide in plain sight. Finding them requires looking.

The Scope of the Problem

Mood Disorders in youth are paradoxical: widespread yet under-recognized, loud yet frequently misheard, clinically visible yet diagnostically obscured by developmental noise, family dynamics, and professional hesitation. Despite decades of evidence, many clinicians still struggle to acknowledge that children—from preschoolers to adolescents—can and do suffer from bipolar spectrum conditions, or what might more accurately be called Mood Disorders of varying intensity and pattern.

This struggle has consequences. Mood Disorder in youth is

missed more often than it is diagnosed, even more frequently than in adults. When unseen, it leaves children misdiagnosed, mistreated, misunderstood— sometimes medicated with antidepressants that destabilize their symptoms— and often discouraged from seeking help again.

The typical trajectory of a young person with an unrecognized Mood Disorder follows a painful pattern. Symptoms emerge in childhood, often before school age. Parents seek help and receive reassurance, or a diagnosis that captures part of the picture but misses the core. Treatment based on the incomplete diagnosis provides partial relief at best, worsening at worst. As the child grows, symptoms evolve but are not resolved. Adolescence brings crisis—academic failure, social collapse, self-harm, hospitalization. Only then, sometimes, does accurate diagnosis occur. But by that point, years have been lost, and the young person's relationship with treatment has often been poisoned by experiences of being misunderstood.

This trajectory is not inevitable. When approached with clinical objectivity, developmental curiosity, and genuine commitment to understanding the child's experience, Mood Disorders become easier to recognize and far more treatable.

This chapter is built on those recognitions—on the lived experiences of young people, the subtleties of differential diagnosis, and the real complexity of treating multi-generational patterns that shape and sometimes destabilize treatment.

EARLY CLUES: Childhood Expressions of Mood Instability

Mood Disorders do not wait for puberty. They announce themselves early—sometimes dramatically—in ways that mimic temperament, behavioral issues, or parenting challenges.

Common early childhood signs include minimal sleep accompanied by bursts of relentless energy, sensory oversensitivity as if emotions strike without filters, tantrums far beyond developmental expectations, sudden shifts from exuberance to despair, anxiety that blends into agitation, and emotional intensity that consumes the child and everyone around them.

Children do not describe mood states—they act them out. What adults interpret as willfulness or defiance may instead be a nervous system out of sync, unable to moderate internal storms. The four-year-old who sleeps three hours and oscillates between ecstatic play and volcanic meltdowns is not simply "difficult." The six-year-old whose rages seem to come from nowhere and vanish just as mysteriously is not merely "strong-willed." These children are experiencing something their developing brains cannot yet name or regulate.

The clinical challenge lies in distinguishing developmental variation from pathology. All young children have limited emotional regulation; all toddlers tantrum; all preschoolers cycle between joy and frustration. But there are children whose intensity, duration, and pattern of emotional dysregulation falls outside developmental norms—children whose internal experience is one of constant storm, who exhaust themselves and their families, who cannot be soothed by ordinary parenting because the fire within burns too hot.

Recognizing early Mood Disorder requires listening not just to symptoms but to severity and pattern. The child whose sleep is consistently and dramatically reduced without daytime fatigue, whose energy surges independent of circumstances, whose emotional shifts occur spontaneously rather than in response to triggers—this child warrants careful evaluation rather than reassurance that they will "grow out of it."

The developmental presentation differs from adult mania in

important ways. Grandiosity in a young child may appear as bossiness, insistence on being in charge, refusal to accept adult authority —behaviors that could be attributed to temperament or parenting but that in context suggest something more. Decreased need for sleep may be attributed to "he's always been a bad sleeper" without recognition that the child is not merely sleeping poorly but is energized rather than fatigued by sleep deprivation. Racing thoughts may manifest as rapid, pressured speech that adults interpret as talkativeness or hyperactivity.

The key is pattern recognition across multiple domains. A single symptom proves little. But when reduced sleep, elevated energy, emotional intensity, and behavioral dysregulation cluster together— and when they occur in episodes rather than as stable traits—the picture of early Mood Disorder begins to emerge.

Adolescence: When Mood Gains a Voice

Adolescence brings language. The child who once erupted now expresses the chaos inside.

"I overthink everything."

"My emotions explode before I can stop them."

"I sleep two hours and feel wired."

"Small things feel like disasters."

Adolescents live with internal conflict layered on developmental turbulence: identity formation, peer pressure, school expectations, early intimacy, and an awareness that something inside them feels different. They compare themselves to peers who seem to navigate emotion with ease, and they wonder what is wrong with them.

They often describe themselves as overwhelmed, raw, eruptive, ashamed, and exhausted from trying to function while managing invisible instability. They develop elaborate strategies to hide their suffering—performing normalcy at school while falling apart at home, or conversely, holding together for parents while unraveling among peers. The energy required for this performance depletes them further.

The metaphor that resonates most with many adolescents is that of rope walkers in a circus—straining for balance, aware that one gust of emotional wind may send them over the edge. They are managing a constant internal negotiation that others cannot see, and they are tired.

Adolescent presentations differ from both childhood and adult presentations in characteristic ways. The mood episodes may be shorter and more frequent than in adults—cycling over days or weeks rather than months. Irritability is often more prominent than euphoria; the "manic" adolescent may be explosively angry rather than expansively happy. Mixed states, in which depressive and hypomanic symptoms occur simultaneously, are common and particularly distressing.

When adolescents are invited to paint their picture of suffering, the alliance begins. They feel seen. And diagnosis moves from a label to a shared understanding. The clinician who asks, "What is it like inside your mind?" rather than checking symptoms off a list often receives answers that clarify everything.

This invitation to self-description serves diagnostic and therapeutic purposes simultaneously. Diagnostically, it elicits information that structured interviews may miss—the subjective quality of racing thoughts, the felt sense of being driven by energy that cannot be controlled, the experience of emotions as overwhelming forces rather than manageable states. Therapeutically, it communicates that the clinician is interested in the adolescent as a person, not merely as a collection of symptoms to be catalogued.

· · ·

WHY MOOD DISORDERS in Youth Are Missed

Despite visible symptoms, Mood Disorders in youth often go undiagnosed. Understanding why illuminates the path toward better recognition.

Adult Diagnostic Bias

Textbook mania and depression rarely appear in children the way they do in adults. Pediatric presentations are developmental, fast-moving, and relational. The grandiosity of a manic adult becomes the bossy, know-it-all quality of a child. The decreased need for sleep becomes a child who "has always been a bad sleeper." The racing thoughts become a child who "can't stop talking" or "jumps from topic to topic." When clinicians look for adult presentations in children, they miss the developmental translations.

Training in adult psychiatry, even when supplemented by child and adolescent rotations, instills templates that may not fit younger patients. The clinician who has learned to recognize mania as euphoric mood, grandiose delusions, and decreased need for sleep over a period of at least one week may not see the irritable, rapid cycling, mixed-state presentation of a twelve-year-old as the same condition.

Misinterpretation of Irritability and Reactivity

Irritability in children can stem from many sources: ADHD, anxiety, trauma, family conflict, learning disabilities, medical illness, or simply being a child in a stressful world. Many clinicians miss attribute mood lability to these causes without considering that it might also—or instead—reflect an underlying Mood Disorder. The child who is "always difficult" or "impossible to please" may be suffering from chronic dysregulation that has a name and a treatment.

Irritability is perhaps the most common symptom of pediatric

Mood Disorders and the most commonly misattributed. Because irritable children are difficult to live with and to treat, irritability itself becomes the focus—something to be managed through behavioral interventions, something that reflects oppositional temperament or inadequate parenting. The possibility that irritability is a mood symptom, arising from the same pathophysiology that produces other mood symptoms, may not be considered.

Professional Hesitation and Stigma

Diagnosing a child with bipolar spectrum illness feels daunting for clinicians and families alike. The label carries weight. It implies lifelong illness, medication, limitation. Clinicians may unconsciously avoid the diagnosis to protect families from this weight—or to protect themselves from difficult conversations. But the consequence of avoiding diagnosis is avoiding treatment, and the child continues to suffer.

The stigma surrounding pediatric bipolar disorder has been intensified by controversies in the field. Debates about whether the condition is overdiagnosed or underdiagnosed, about whether pediatric presentations truly represent the same disorder as adult bipolar disorder, and about the appropriateness of psychotropic medication in children have created an atmosphere of caution that sometimes tips into avoidance. Clinicians who are uncertain may choose not to diagnose rather than risk being wrong.

Yet the cost of underdiagnosis is real and measurable in suffering. The child who does have a Mood Disorder and does not receive treatment continues to cycle, continues to struggle, continues to accumulate the consequences of untreated illness.

Antidepressant Missteps

A child or adolescent presents with depression, low mood, withdrawal, hopelessness. The clinician prescribes an SSRI, following guidelines for pediatric depression. But if the underlying condition is a Mood Disorder with depressive and hypomanic or manic features, the antidepressant may worsen rather than help. Agitation increases, sleep deteriorates further, impulsivity rises, and cycling accelerates. Sometimes self-harm emerges or worsens. The child and family conclude that treatment made things worse, and they withdraw from care—often for years.

This pattern is tragically common. Antidepressant activation in a young person with unrecognized bipolar spectrum disorder can precipitate a crisis that shapes the patient's relationship with treatment for years to come. The experience of being made worse by medication trusting a clinician and being harmed—is not easily overcome.

Prevention requires careful assessment before prescribing antidepressants to any young person presenting with depression. Family history of bipolar disorder, personal history of hypomanic symptoms (even if not previously recognized), and the quality of the depressive episode itself (mixed features, atypical features, psychotic features) should all be evaluated. When bipolar spectrum disorder is possible, mood stabilization should precede or accompany antidepressant treatment.

Family and School Narratives

Adults often describe symptoms as "behavior problems" or "immaturity" rather than as signs of illness. The child is labeled defiant, oppositional, attention-seeking, dramatic, or manipulative. These labels obscure the biological roots of the behavior and direct intervention toward discipline and consequences rather than treatment. By the time the child reaches a clinician, the narrative is set, and it takes deliberate effort to look beneath it.

The narratives that families and schools construct around a

child's difficulties are not arbitrary; they represent attempts to make sense of puzzling and distressing behavior. But once established, these narratives filter subsequent observations. The teacher who has decided that a child is "manipulative" interprets mood-driven behavior through that lens. The parent who has concluded that the child "just needs more discipline" seeks behavioral rather than psychiatric intervention.

The clinician's task is to hold existing narratives lightly while gathering information that may support or contradict them. Sometimes the narrative is correct; sometimes it captures part of the truth; sometimes it obscures what is actually happening. Careful history-taking that asks about symptom patterns, episodicity, and neurovegetative features can reveal the mood disorder that behavior-focused narratives have hidden.

HERITABILITY: A Family Story Across Generations

Mood Disorders are among the most heritable psychiatric conditions. Genetics are complex—no single gene determines outcome—but the familial clustering is unmistakable. In practice, it is common to treat two generations, often three, occasionally four.

Patterns echo down family lines: the same sensitivities, the same storms, the same collapses, and, importantly, the same potential for recovery. The grandmother who was "always moody" and self-medicated with alcohol. The father whose career was derailed by episodes he never understood. The mother, who finally received diagnosis and treatment in her thirties and now watches her children showing early signs. The child who carries the family vulnerability into a new generation.

Recognizing this generational thread often brings enormous

relief. Families have typically spent years wondering what went wrong—blaming parenting, blaming circumstances, blaming themselves. When they learn that what they are dealing with is biological, heritable, and treatable, something shifts.

"It wasn't my fault. This runs in our family. Now we understand."

This understanding does not minimize the difficulty ahead, but it redirects energy from blame to treatment. Parents who blame themselves for their child's struggles can instead become partners in care. Children who believe they were fundamentally flawed can instead understand themselves as having a condition— something that is part of them but not all of them, something that can be managed.

The heritability of Mood Disorders also has practical clinical implications. Family history of bipolar disorder, especially with response to particular medications, can guide treatment choices. When a parent has responded well to a specific mood stabilizer, the child often responds to the same medication. This is not universal, but it is common enough to inform clinical decision-making.

Taking a careful family history is therefore essential in evaluating any child or adolescent for possible Mood Disorder. The history should include not just formal diagnoses but functional descriptions: relatives who had "bad tempers" or "mood swings," who were hospitalized psychiatrically, who had problems with alcohol or drugs, who died by suicide, who had periods of high productivity followed by collapses, who were described as "too sensitive" or "too intense." These descriptions often point toward mood disorders that were never formally diagnosed.

A CENTRAL VIGNETTE: Two Generations and the Fragility of Stability

A fifteen-year-old girl was brought in by her mother, who was already my patient. The mother had responded well to Lamotrigine and Lurasidone, stabilizing after years of turbulent mood and missing diagnosis. Now she was worried about her daughter.

The girl carried a painful history of missed diagnosis as well.

One year earlier, she had been hospitalized and diagnosed with Major Depressive Disorder. She was prescribed an antidepressant. But she worsened—sleep decreased, agitation rose, self-harm emerged. The antidepressant had destabilized her, activating the hypomanic potential that no one had recognized. Feeling misunderstood and hopeless, she dropped out of treatment entirely.

Now she came with mood swings, reduced sleep with intermittent high energy, superficial cutting once or twice a month, overwhelming overthinking, emotional overreactions she could not contain, failing grades, and retreating from friends and a budding romantic relationship.

When I asked what she most wanted from treatment, her priority was deeply human: "I want my social life back."

I told her: "Let's help you rebuild the parts of life you care about. That is our work together."

Given her symptoms and her mother's treatment response, I prescribed the same combination that had helped her mother. She improved quickly. Friendships stabilized. Grades rose. Emotional storms quieted. Self-harm ceased. She began to recognize herself again.

Soon her seventeen-year-old brother was referred. He was also diagnosed with a Mood Disorder, complicated by ADHD. With treatment, he flourished as well.

For a moment, the family healed.

The mother, now stable for the first time in years, began working an extra job to save money for her children's future. It was an act of love—she wanted to give them opportunities she had missed during her own years of untreated illness.

But her increased absence left her daughter feeling unanchored. The connection that had supported treatment frayed. Quietly, without anger or intention to rebel, the girl stopped her medications. She did not tell anyone. Within weeks, her symptoms returned.

Lessons from the Vignette

This vignette reveals clinical truths that no manual teaches.

Mood Disorders run through families—not just biologically, but emotionally. The patterns that shape one generation's experience influence the next. The mother's illness had shaped the daughter's childhood; the mother's recovery had made the daughter's treatment possible.

Family dynamics can stabilize or destabilize treatment. The mother's new job was motivated by care for her children, but its practical effect was reduced availability, and for a teenager whose stability depended partly on maternal connection, this was destabilizing.

Even successful treatment is fragile without sustained support. The daughter had responded beautifully to medication. But medication alone, without the relational context that supported adherence and gave meaning to recovery, proved insufficient.

Adherence is relational, not simply behavioral. Patients do not stop medication because they forget or because they are irresponsible. They stop because medication exists within a web of meaning, relationship, and circumstance. When that web frays, adherence becomes harder.

Misdiagnosis and antidepressant missteps can derail a young life. The daughter's first encounter with treatment was harmful. She was given medication that made her worse, and she concluded—reasonably—that treatment was dangerous. It took a year and her mother's example to bring her back to care.

This family's story is not uncommon. It is the reason this chapter exists.

ADDITIONAL VIGNETTES

Early Childhood: The Storm Before Language

A four-year-old boy arrived gripping a worn dinosaur toy. His parents, exhausted and bewildered, described a child who had never slept more than three or four hours a night—not from birth, not ever. He cycled between ecstatic, creative play that could last for hours and volcanic tantrums that seemed to come from nowhere and could not be soothed by any ordinary means.

His parents had tried everything. Consistent routines, Consequences, and rewards. Parenting classes, Occupational therapy; nothing had helped. They had been told he was willful, that they were too permissive, that he would grow out of it.

But this was not naughtiness or the result of poor parenting. This was early Mood Disorder—unfiltered, pre-verbal, overwhelming. His nervous system was running too fast, generating more energy than his small body could manage, cycling through states that he could not name or understand.

Treatment brought relief that the family had stopped hoping for. His sleep improved. The tantrums became less frequent and less intense. He began to engage with preschool, to make friends, to show the sweet nature that had always been there but had been obscured by storms.

His parents wept when they saw the change. "We have our son back," they said. But he had never been gone— only hidden beneath symptoms that no one had recognized.

The High-Functioning Teen: Brilliance at a Cost

A sixteen-year-old girl was referred by her school counselor, who was concerned about what she called "perfectionism taken too far."

The girl excelled academically—near the top of her class, multiple AP courses, leadership positions in clubs, volunteer work that filled every remaining hour. But the counselor had noticed that her involvement was not steady. She would take on multiple new commitments in bursts of enthusiasm, work on them intensely for weeks, then withdraw suddenly, citing exhaustion or overwhelm. Then the cycle would repeat.

In my office, the girl described her inner experience: she slept four hours a night and felt fine—more than fine, she felt alive and powerful during those periods. Her mind raced with ideas and plans. She joined activities impulsively; certain she could handle anything. Then something would shift. She would collapse emotionally, sleep for days, miss school, feel hopeless and empty. The cycle took weeks to months.

Teachers saw perfectionism. They saw a high-achieving student who sometimes pushed too hard. They did not see the silent torment:

"My brain doesn't rest until it shuts down. I don't know how to explain it. It's like I'm running a race that never ends, and then suddenly I can't take another step."

Diagnosis gave her permission to breathe. It explained what she had been experiencing. It offered a path toward stability that did not require giving up her ambitions but did require learning to work with her brain rather than against it.

Severe Case: When Safety Must Lead

A seventeen-year-old boy was brought to the emergency department after running barefoot into the night, convinced he was receiving messages from a source he could not name. He had not slept in four days. He was speaking rapidly, connecting ideas that made sense only to him, laughing at things no one else found funny.

This was mania with psychotic features—unmistakable, severe, dangerous. He could not keep himself safe. Hospitalization was necessary.

On the unit, with medication and containment, he gradually returned to himself. The racing thoughts slowed. Sleep returned. The delusional beliefs faded. In his first coherent conversation, he said: "It felt like my brain had left me."

It hadn't. It simply needed help.

His recovery was not simple. He grieved the experience, felt ashamed of what he had done while manic, worried about what it meant for his future. But with treatment and support, he graduated high school, enrolled in college, and learned to manage a condition that had briefly taken over his life.

Not every severe case ends this well. But many do when treatment is adequate and sustained.

DIFFERENTIAL DIAGNOSIS: **Distinguishing Mood Disorders from Look-Alikes**

Several conditions share features with Mood Disorders in youth, and careful differential diagnosis is essential. The following sections address the most common sources of diagnostic confusion.

ADHD and Mood Disorders

ADHD and Mood Disorders frequently co-occur, and their symptoms overlap in ways that complicate diagnosis. Both involve impulsivity, restlessness, difficulty concentrating, and emotional reactivity.

The key distinguishing features relate to course, sleep, and treatment response. ADHD symptoms are chronic and consistent—the child has always been this way, in all settings, without periods of marked worsening or improvement unrelated to circumstances. Mood Disorder symptoms are episodic— there are better periods and worse periods, even if the baseline is abnormal.

Sleep patterns differ characteristically. The child with ADHD who sleeps poorly is tired; the child with hypomania who sleeps poorly is energized. This distinction is clinically important and often overlooked.

Treatment response provides additional information. Stimulant medications typically help ADHD symptoms without causing mood destabilization. In a child with an unrecognized Mood Disorder, stimulants may worsen mood symptoms, increase irritability and agitation, or precipitate a more clearly hypomanic or manic state.

Many children have both conditions, and both require treatment. The general principle is to stabilize mood first, then address ADHD, as treating ADHD in the context of unstable mood often makes everything worse.

Anxiety and Mood Disorders

Anxiety is nearly universal in Mood Disorders— it may be the most common symptom. Children with Mood Disorders overthink, worry, feel on edge, have physical symptoms of anxiety, and often meet criteria for anxiety disorders.

The distinguishing features relate to the presence of mood episodes. The child with an anxiety disorder is chronically anxious without episodes of reduced need for sleep, elevated energy, or expanded mood. The child with a Mood Disorder has anxiety plus episodic changes in energy, sleep, and activation that go beyond anxious arousal.

Treatment implications follow from accurate diagnosis. Anxiety in the context of a Mood Disorder often improves with mood stabilization; treating only anxiety with SSRIs may destabilize the mood.

Trauma and Mood Disorders

Trauma can cause mood instability, emotional reactivity, and cycling between emotional states. In some children, what appears to be a Mood Disorder is actually a trauma response.

The distinguishing features relate to triggers and pattern. Trauma-related symptoms are typically linked to reminders of the traumatic experience—certain situations, people, sensory stimuli, or times of year. Mood Disorder symptoms cycle spontaneously, independent of external triggers.

Many children have both trauma histories and Mood Disorders. The trauma may have been both cause and consequence— cause because early adversity can influence brain development in ways that increase mood vulnerability, consequence because children with Mood Disorders are more likely to experience traumatic events due to impulsivity, poor judgment during episodes, or family dysfunction related to parental illness.

When both are present, both require attention. Trauma-focused treatment may be necessary alongside mood stabilization.

Disruptive Mood Dysregulation Disorder

DMDD was introduced as a diagnostic category partly to address concerns about overdiagnosis of bipolar disorder in children. It describes children with severe, chronic irritability and frequent temper outbursts.

The distinguishing feature is the absence of distinct episodes. DMDD is characterized by chronic irritability without hypomanic or manic periods. The child is irritable essentially all the time, not cycling between irritable and non-irritable states.

In practice, the distinction is not always clear. Some children with DMDD may have a Mood Disorder that presents primarily with irritability; some children diagnosed with pediatric bipolar disorder may be better characterized as having DMDD. Careful longitudinal observation often clarifies the picture over time.

Substance Use

In adolescents, substance use can cause mood symptoms that mimic Mood Disorders. Intoxication, withdrawal, and the chaos of substance-affected life all contribute to emotional instability.

The distinguishing feature is temporal relationship. Mood symptoms that emerge only during active substance use and resolve with abstinence are likely substance-induced rather than indicating a primary Mood Disorder. However, many adolescents with Mood Disorders use substances to self-medicate, and the two conditions often co-occur.

Differential Diagnosis at a Glance

The following table summarizes the key distinguishing features of conditions commonly confused with Mood Disorders in youth.

Condition	Overlapping Features	Distinguishing Features
ADHD	Impulsivity, restlessness, poor concentration	Symptoms chronic and stable, not episodic; sleep loss causes fatigue rather than energy
Anxiety	Overthinking, irritability, agitation	No episodic decreased need for sleep or elevated energy; anxiety is persistent rather than cycling
Trauma/PTSD	Emotional reactivity, mood swings, dysregulation	Symptoms tied to trauma triggers; lacks spontaneous cycling unrelated to reminders
DMDD	Severe irritability, temper outbursts	Chronic irritability without discrete hypomanic or manic periods
Substance Use	Mood swings, agitation, impulsivity	Temporally linked to substance use; symptoms resolve with sustained abstinence

ADHD vs. Bipolar Spectrum: A Clarifying Comparison

Because ADHD and bipolar spectrum disorders so frequently co-occur and share surface features, direct comparison is particularly useful for clinicians.

Feature	ADHD	Bipolar Spectrum
Course	Stable and chronic	Episodic with periods of worsening and improvement
Sleep	Poor sleep leads to fatigue and worsened functioning	Reduced sleep occurs without fatigue; child is energized
Energy	Restless, fidgety, needs to move	Episodically elevated; doing more than usual
Thought	Distractible; attention pulled by stimuli	Racing; ideas come too fast; pressured speech
Impulsivity	Chronic and consistent across time	Worsens during mood episodes compared to baseline
Response to Stimulants	Typically helpful for core symptoms	May destabilize mood if bipolar is untreated

Distinguishing Features

ADHD

Impulsivity, restlessness, poor concentration

Symptoms chronic and stable, not episodic; sleep loss causes fatigue rather than energy

Anxiety

Overthinking, irritability, agitation

No episodic decreased need for sleep or elevated energy; anxiety is persistent rather than cycling

Trauma/PTSD

Emotional reactivity, mood swings, dysregulation

Symptoms tied to trauma triggers; lacks spontaneous cycling unrelated to reminders

DMDD

Severe irritability, temper outbursts

Chronic irritability without discrete hypomanic or manic periods

Substance Use

Mood swings, agitation, impulsivity

Temporally linked to substance use; symptoms resolve with sustained abstinence

ADHD VS. BIPOLAR SPECTRUM: A Clarifying Comparison

Because ADHD and bipolar spectrum disorders so frequently co-occur and share surface features, direct comparison is particularly useful for clinicians.

Overlapping features

ADHD Vs Bipolar Spectrum

Course

Stable and chronic Vs episodic with periods of worsening and improvement

Sleep

Poor sleep leads to fatigue and worsened functioning Vs Reduced sleep occurs without fatigue; child is energized

Energy

Restless, fidgety, needs to move Vs Episodically elevated; doing more than usual

Thought

Distractible; attention pulled by stimuli Vs Racing; ideas come too fast; pressured speech

Impulsivity

Chronic and consistent across time Vs Worsens during mood episodes compared to baseline

Response to Stimulants

Typically helpful for core symptoms Vs May destabilize mood if bipolar is untreated

The practical implication is that when both conditions are suspected, mood stabilization should generally precede stimulant treatment. Starting stimulants in a child with active mood instability often worsens the overall picture. Once mood is stable, ADHD can be addressed, and stimulants are often well-tolerated at that point.

TREATMENT CONSIDERATIONS

Treatment of Mood Disorders in youth requires integration of pharmacological and non-pharmacological approaches, attention to family dynamics, and patience with the process of finding optimal medication.

Pharmacological Treatment

The evidence base for pharmacological treatment of pediatric Mood Disorders continues to develop. Mood stabilizers, atypical antipsychotics, and combinations of these agents are the mainstays of treatment. The choice of agent depends on symptom profile, family history of medication response, comorbidities, and practical considerations like monitoring requirements.

Starting doses should be low and titration gradual. Children and adolescents are often more sensitive to medication effects than adults, and tolerability determines adherence. The medication that works in theory but causes intolerable side effects in practice is not useful.

Family history of medications response provides valuable guidance. When a parent has responded well to a specific mood stabilizer, the child often responds to the same medication. This pattern, while not universal, is common enough to inform initial treatment selection.

The danger of antidepressant monotherapy in youth with Mood

Disorders warrants repeated emphasis. Antidepressants can destabi-lize mood, increase cycling, worsen agitation and impulsivity, and precipitate frank mania. When depression is prominent in a young person with known or suspected Mood Disorder, treatment with a mood stabilizer first—with antidepressant added cautiously later if needed—is generally safer than antidepressant monotherapy.

Psychotherapy

Psychotherapy plays essential roles in treatment of youth with Mood Disorders, complementing pharmacological intervention.

Psychoeducation helps young people and families understand what they are dealing with. Knowledge about the condition—its biological basis, its typical course, its treatability—reduces blame and shame while increasing engagement with treatment.

Skill building provides tools for mood monitoring, trigger recog-nition, and early intervention when symptoms begin to escalate. Adolescents who can identify the early signs of a mood episode and take protective action—adjusting sleep, reducing stimulation, reaching out for help—have better outcomes than those who are blindsided by each episode.

Addressing psychological consequences is necessary because living with a mood disorder has psychological effects beyond the symptoms themselves. Young people may carry shame about their illness, grief about the life they imagined, disrupted identity develop-ment, or damaged relationships that need repair.

Family therapy or family involvement improves outcomes in most cases. Parents who understand the condition, who can monitor symptoms between visits, who can support adherence, and who can maintain their own stability provide a foundation for their child's recovery.

Specific modalities with evidence in pediatric populations include family-focused therapy, interpersonal and social rhythm therapy adapted for adolescents, and cognitive-behavioral approaches. The specific modality may matter less than the presence of a consistent, supportive therapeutic relationship.

Family Involvement

Because Mood Disorders are heritable, treatment often occurs in a family context where other members are also affected. Parents with their own mood disorders may struggle to provide the stability their children need. Siblings may be symptomatic or may be bearing burdens of caregiving beyond their years. Family patterns that developed around untreated illness may persist even after treatment begins.

Family involvement in treatment—whether through family therapy, parent training, or simply including parents in medication visits —typically improves outcomes. The family is not merely the context in which treatment occurs; the family is part of the treatment.

Sometimes family dynamics actively undermine treatment. A parent whose own mood disorder is untreated may sabotage the child's treatment, either unconsciously or through explicit interference. Marital conflict may destabilize the child regardless of medication. In these situations, addressing family factors becomes essential —not as a replacement for the child's treatment but as a necessary complement to it.

School Involvement

Academic functioning is nearly always affected by Mood Disorders in youth. Episodes disrupt attendance, concentration, and motivation. The chronic effort of managing symptoms depletes energy that would otherwise go to learning. Relationships with peers and teachers suffer during symptomatic periods.

Schools can provide accommodations that support functioning during periods of instability—extended time on assignments, flexibility with attendance, modified workloads during acute episodes, access to a counselor or quiet space when needed. These accommodations are not special privileges; they are recognition that the student is managing a medical condition that affects functioning.

Collaboration between clinicians, families, and schools often requires explicit attention; it does not happen automatically. Parents may need guidance on how to communicate with schools about their child's needs without disclosing more than necessary. Schools may need education about mood disorders and their impact on learning. Clinicians may need to provide documentation or participate in meetings.

When school involvement works well, it extends the treatment into the environment where the child spends most of their waking hours. When it fails, the child faces the challenge of managing illness while also managing an unsupportive or punitive school environment.

LONG-TERM PERSPECTIVE

Mood Disorders that begin in childhood or adolescence are typically lifelong conditions requiring ongoing management. This is hard news for young people and families who may hope that treatment will constitute a cure.

Yet the long-term perspective also offers hope. Many young people with Mood Disorders go on to live full, meaningful lives—completing education, building careers, forming relationships, raising families. The condition shapes their lives but does not determine them.

Early diagnosis and treatment may improve long-term prognosis. Children and adolescents who receive appropriate treatment develop skills for managing their condition that serve them throughout life.

They avoid years of misdiagnosis, ineffective treatment, and accumulated consequences of untreated illness.

The relationship between clinician and youth often sets the template for the patient's relationship with treatment throughout life. The young person who experiences treatment as helpful, respectful, and collaborative develops expectations that they will bring to future care. The young person whose first treatment experience is negative — who was misunderstood, given harmful medication, or blamed for their symptoms—may avoid treatment for years or decades.

This responsibility should weigh on every clinician who treats mood disorders in young people. We are not only treating the current episode; we are shaping the patient's relationship with treatment for life.

Transitions in care deserve particular attention. The adolescent who has been treated successfully by a child psychiatrist will eventually age out of that practice. The transition to adult care is a vulnerable period when continuity may be lost and adherence may lapse. Planning for this transition, making warm handoffs when possible, and ensuring that treatment history is communicated to new providers can protect the gains that have been made.

CONCLUSION: **Seeing and Hearing**

The title of this chapter—"Seeing the Unseen, Hearing the Unsaid"—captures the clinical task.

Mood Disorders in youth are unseen because their presentations do not match adult templates, because they hide behind behavioral labels, because clinicians and families alike resist the diagnosis. The clinician who sees Mood Disorder must look beneath surface presentations, consider developmental translations of adult symptoms, and tolerate the discomfort of making a diagnosis that carries weight.

Mood Disorders in youth are unsaid because children lack language for their internal experiences, because adolescents have learned to hide their struggles, because families frame symptoms in terms that obscure their meaning. The clinician who hears the unsaid must invite young people to describe their inner world, must listen for what is implied rather than stated, must help patients find words for experiences that have felt nameless.

When we see and hear accurately, diagnosis becomes possible. When diagnosis is accurate, treatment can begin. When treatment is appropriate and sustained, lives change.

The four-year-old clutching his dinosaur can grow into a child who sleeps, who plays without volcanic eruptions, who engages with school and peers. The fifteen-year-old who stopped treatment after antidepressants made her worse can find medication that helps and rebuild her social life. The seventeen-year-old who ran barefoot into the night can return to himself and build a future.

These outcomes are possible. They require clinicians willing to see what others have missed and hear what has not been spoken or heard.

KEY POINTS for Patients and Families

Mood Disorders can begin in early childhood— they do not wait for adolescence or adulthood. If your child has always seemed "different" in their intensity, sleep patterns, or emotional storms, this warrants evaluation.

Misdiagnosis is common. If your child has been diagnosed with ADHD, anxiety, or behavioral problems but treatment has not helped, or if antidepressants have made things worse, consider whether an underlying Mood Disorder might have been missed.

Family history matters. If mood disorders, bipolar disorder, or related conditions run in your family, your child may carry the same vulnerability. This is not your fault, and knowing about it can guide treatment.

Accurate diagnosis brings relief. Understanding that your child has a biological condition—not a character flaw or the result of bad parenting—allows everyone to redirect energy from blame to treatment.

Treatment works for most young people with Mood Disorders. It may take time to find the right medication, and medication is usually not the only component of treatment, but improvement is the expected outcome.

Be wary of antidepressant monotherapy. If your child or adolescent with mood instability is prescribed an antidepressant alone, ask the prescriber about the possibility of bipolar spectrum disorder and whether a mood stabilizer should be considered.

Stay involved in treatment. Your observations about your child's symptoms, your support for medication adherence, and your maintenance of a stable home environment all contribute to your child's recovery.

The goal is not just symptom control but a life worth living. Treatment should help your child return to friendships, school, activities, and the developmental tasks of growing up.

QUESTIONS FOR REFLECTION and Discussion

1. How do developmental factors change the presentation of Mood Disorders in children compared to adults?
2. Why might a clinician hesitate to diagnose bipolar spectrum disorder in a child, and what are the consequences of this hesitation?

3. What role does family history play in both the development and treatment of Mood Disorders in youth?

4. How can clinicians distinguish between ADHD and bipolar spectrum disorder when both involve impulsivity and hyperactivity?

5. What are the risks of prescribing antidepressant monotherapy to a young person with an unrecognized Mood Disorder?

6. How do family dynamics influence treatment adherence and outcomes in adolescents with Mood Disorders?

7. What does "seeing the unseen and hearing the unsaid" mean in the context of diagnosing Mood Disorders in youth?

SUMMARY

Mood Disorders in childhood and adolescence are common, heritable, and treatable—yet they remain underdiagnosed. This chapter has examined the reasons for diagnostic failure, the developmental presentations that differ from adult templates, the conditions that mimic or co-occur with Mood Disorders, and the principles of treatment.

The central argument is simple: clinicians must be willing to look for Mood Disorders in young people rather than waiting for unmistakable adult-type presentations. They must ask the questions that elicit the unsaid—the internal experiences that young people cannot articulate without invitation. They must tolerate the weight of making a diagnosis that has lifelong implications, recognizing that the alternative—missed diagnosis—has consequences that are often worse.

When diagnosis is accurate and treatment is appropriate, outcomes are often good. Young people with Mood Disorders can learn to manage their conditions, can complete their developmental tasks, can build lives of meaning and connection. This is the goal of treatment and the reason this chapter exists.

6

PSYCHOPHARMACOLOGY
IN YOUNG ADULTHOOD

Young adulthood is a crossing— a liminal space between the scaffolding of adolescence and the first true steps into independent life. In this transition, everything is in motion: identity, relationships, values, ambitions, bodies, brains, and the meaning of illness itself. Psychopharmacology in this stage is both an opportunity and a delicate responsibility.

Young adults stand at the confluence of freedom and vulnerability. They are negotiating the loss of structure, the acquisition of autonomy, and the pressure to discover who they are and where they are going. Symptoms that began quietly in childhood or adolescence may surge during this period. Some diagnoses crystallize; others blur. Medication decisions become personal rather than parent-driven, yet not always wisely guided.

Treating young adults requires a clinician to understand the developmental turbulence beneath the symptoms: the struggle between separation and belonging, responsibility and avoidance, aspiration, and fear.

. . .

I. THE DEVELOPMENTAL LANDSCAPE: **The Brain Still Becoming**

Although young adults appear physically mature, the prefrontal cortex continues developing well into the late twenties. Executive functioning—planning, impulse control, organization, time perception—remains incomplete. This asymmetry between apparent maturity and neurobiological reality makes the transition to adulthood particularly challenging.

Young adults often face unsupervised schedules for the first time, along with academic or workplace demands that exceed anything previously encountered. Financial stress compounds these pressures. Many experience loneliness or instability in relationships as they leave the social structures of high school or their family home. Sleep patterns become disrupted, sometimes severely. Exposure to alcohol and substances increases dramatically in environments with minimal oversight.

Symptoms worsen during this period not because young adults are irresponsible, but because they are still becoming—and this becoming is taxing. The clinician who attributes deterioration to character flaws misses the developmental reality. The one who recognizes the strain of this transition can offer both understanding and practical support.

II. **The Meaning of Medication Shifts**

In adolescence, medication is often guided—or imposed—by adults. Parents manage prescriptions, monitor adherence, and make decisions that adolescents may accept, resist, or simply tolerate. For young adults, taking medication raises identity issues.

Young adults ask themselves whether they want medication to be part of their story. They wonder whether medication will change who they are at some fundamental level. They question whether needing help means they are flawed. They grapple with whether their condition is temporary or a lifelong reality they must accept.

Some reject medication as an act of independence, proving to themselves and others that they can manage without pharmaceutical support. Others cling to medication as a lifeline, fearful of what might happen without it. Many oscillate, stopping and restarting in cycles that mirror their emotional tides and shifting self-concepts.

The clinician's task is to help the young adult reframe medication as a tool rather than an identity, a bridge to the life they want rather than a symbol of limitation. This reframing cannot be imposed; it must emerge through relationship, conversation, and the young adult's own reflection.

III. When Diagnosis Comes Into Focus

Young adulthood is a time when many psychiatric disorders emerge or reveal their full expression. The clinician must be prepared for diagnostic complexity and evolution.

Mood disorders often intensify during this period. Stress, irregular sleep, and new freedoms can trigger bipolar or depressive episodes that may have been muted or manageable during adolescence. The first clear manic episode frequently occurs during college years or shortly after, often precipitated by sleep deprivation, substance use, or the loss of family structure.

Psychotic disorders commonly declare themselves during late adolescence through the mid-twenties. This developmental window represents the peak period for first psychotic breaks. Early and effective treatment during this critical period profoundly alters long-term outcomes—a reality that makes timely intervention particularly consequential.

Anxiety disorders often come to the forefront when young adults face high-pressure environments, significant transitions, and identity uncertainty. Social anxiety that was manageable in familiar settings may become debilitating in new social contexts. Generalized anxiety may surge when the predictable structures of earlier life disappear.

ADHD and executive dysfunction often become truly debilitating for the first time in young adulthood. Previously, these difficulties may have been masked by parental structure, academic scaffolding, or the shorter time horizons of earlier developmental stages. When these supports disappear with an increase in demands put upon this population, executive dysfunction can derail academic performance, employment, and relationships.

Substance use disorders complicate nearly every aspect of diagnosis and treatment. Alcohol, cannabis, non-prescribed stimulants, psychedelics, and vaping all alter symptom presentation, interact with medications, and confound clinical assessment. Treating psychiatric disorders requires addressing substance use, just as effective substance use intervention demands attention to underlying psychiatric issues.

Diagnosis in young adulthood requires patience, developmental understanding, and curiosity about the whole person—not just the presenting symptom. What appears to be one disorder may evolve into another. What seems like substance-induced psychosis may herald schizophrenia. What presents as depression may be the depressive pole of bipolar disorder. The clinician must hold diagnoses tentatively, remain alert to evolution, and communicate uncertainty honestly.

. . .

IV. The Therapeutic Alliance Reimagined

Treating young adults requires respecting autonomy while offering steady guidance. The clinician must avoid both paternalism and passivity. Paternalism—treating the young adult as a larger adolescent who needs direction—provokes resistance and undermines the developmental task of claiming one's own life. Passivity—refusing to offer guidance because the young adult is technically an adult—abandons someone who still needs mentorship even while asserting independence.

A wise therapeutic stance emphasizes collaboration rather than direction. It honors ambivalence as a normal feature of this developmental period rather than treating it as pathology or resistance. It explores the meaning of medication and symptoms rather than enforcing compliance through pressure or guilt. It invites agency, even in medication decisions; recognizing that young adults who participate in their treatment are more likely to sustain it.

Conversations often shift during young adulthood from symptom reduction toward life-building. The clinician might ask who the young adult is becoming, what obstacles stand in the way of that becoming, and how treatment might support goals the young adult has defined for themselves. In this frame, medication becomes a component of self-authorship rather than a submission to medical authority.

V. Adherence: Freedom's Double-Edged Sword

Once young adults leave home, adherence frequently deteriorates. This is rarely simple rebellion. Routines that previously supported medication-taking collapse. Refills are forgotten amid the chaos of new responsibilities. Pharmacies change when young adults move, and relationships with familiar pharmacists disappear. Insurance lapses during transitions between parental coverage and independent plans. Stigma grows when peers know nothing of childhood diagnoses. Substances interfere with both motivation and memory. Symptoms themselves distort insight, making medication seem unnecessary precisely when it is most needed.

Supporting adherence in young adulthood requires practical strategies rather than lectures. Simplifying regimens helps—a single daily medication is more likely to be taken than a complex multi-dose schedule. Engaging support networks, with the young adult's consent, provides backup when self-monitoring fails. Planning explicitly for transitions—moves, job changes, insurance shifts—prevents predictable lapses. Integrating reminders and technology, such as phone alarms or pill-tracking apps, compensates for executive dysfunction. Offering predictable follow-up creates accountability that the young adult can rely upon even when internal motivation wavers.

The goal is continuity, not perfection. The clinician who expects flawless adherence will be perpetually disappointed; the one who expects imperfection and plans for it will be more helpful.

VI. Family Roles in Transition

Parents remain emotionally invested in their young adult children but must renegotiate boundaries that were clearer during childhood and adolescence. They often struggle to know when support becomes interference and when stepping back becomes abandonment.

The clinician can help families shift from managing the young adult's treatment to supporting their autonomy. This may involve explicit conversations about what information will be shared, how parents can be helpful without being intrusive, and how the young adult can ask for help without feeling diminished. The goal is a gradual transfer of responsibility that respects the young adult's growing capacity while acknowledging that this capacity is still developing.

Some families navigate this transition gracefully; others require ongoing guidance. The clinician serves as a facilitator of this developmental process, not merely a prescriber of medications.

VII. Medication Strategies in Young Adulthood

Medication in young adulthood is not only pharmacology but also prevention, protection, and the shaping of a life trajectory. Several considerations deserve particular attention.

Early, Effective Treatment Reduces Lifelong Suffering

Severe mental illnesses often declare themselves between ages eighteen and twenty-five. Delays in treatment during this critical window can have enduring effects that compound across the lifespan.

Effective early intervention reduces relapse frequency and severity. It preserves cognitive functioning that might otherwise deteriorate with repeated episodes. It stabilizes identity formation during a period when the self is still consolidating. It supports academic and occupational success by maintaining the functioning necessary to meet developmental milestones. It decreases suicide risk, which peaks during this period for many disorders. It protects the emerging adult from catastrophic derailment—the failed semesters, lost jobs, damaged relationships, and legal problems that can accumulate during untreated illness.

Treatment during young adulthood is not only symptom control —it is trajectory-shaping. The clinician who treats aggressively and effectively during this window may prevent decades of avoidable suffering.

The Essential Role of Long-Acting Injectables

Long-acting injectable medications are transformative in young adulthood precisely because adherence is so fragile during this period.

These medications bypass the daily decision-making that oral medications require. They prevent relapse during chaotic transitions when routines collapse. They stabilize mood and thought even when daily structure disappears. They reduce family conflict about adherence by removing the daily medication battle from the relationship. They protect education, work, and relationships by maintaining stability through turbulent periods. They allow the young adult to step outside daily medication decisions and focus on living rather than managing pills.

Long acting injectables should be framed not as external control but as a form of freedom. The clinician might say something like: "This lets your brain stay steady so you can focus on living your life rather than remembering pills every day."

Using these medications earlier in the illness course—not only after repeated relapses have caused cumulative damage—can prevent years of avoidable suffering. The clinician who waits for multiple hospitalizations before suggesting a long-acting injectable has waited too long.

Alcohol and Substance Use: The Quiet Saboteurs

Substances reshape symptom expression and interfere with virtually all psychiatric medications. Their role must be addressed directly, though without moralism.

Cannabis worsens paranoia, anxiety, and mood dysregulation in vulnerable individuals. Alcohol disrupts sleep architecture and undermines antidepressant efficacy. Stimulants can trigger mania or psychosis in those with bipolar disorder or psychotic vulnerability. Psychedelics destabilize already-vulnerable minds in unpredictable ways.

A compassionate, realistic stance allows these topics to be discussed productively. The clinician might say: "This isn't about judgment. It's about understanding how substances interact with your brain so treatment can actually work." This framing invite honesty rather than provoking defensiveness.

Sleep as a Clinical Intervention

Sleep deprivation in vulnerable young adults is not merely uncomfortable—it is a direct threat to psychiatric stability.

Disrupted sleep precipitates manic episodes in those with bipolar vulnerability. It worsens depression by impairing emotional regulation and amplifying negative cognition. It impairs the cognitive functioning that young adults need for academic and occupational success. It intensifies impulsivity, leading to decisions that create lasting consequences. It interacts dangerously with substances, amplifying intoxication, and impairing judgment. It increases vulnerability to exploitation by compromising the capacity for self-protection.

Restoring sleep is often the most transformative therapeutic act available. Before adding or adjusting psychiatric medications, the clinician should assess sleep thoroughly and address it directly. Sometimes sleep restoration alone produces dramatic improvement; often it is the necessary foundation upon which other interventions can build.

Sexual Vulnerability and Victimization

Young adults—especially young women with unstable mood, substance use, or poor sleep—are disproportionately targeted for predatory sexual behavior. This reality deserves direct clinical attention.

Symptoms of psychiatric illness heighten risk in multiple ways. Impaired judgment during mood episodes compromises decision-making about sexual situations. Loneliness drives connection-seeking that may override caution. Poor boundaries, often a feature of certain personality patterns or trauma histories, make exploitation easier. Desperation for connection leads to tolerance of treatment that would otherwise be rejected. Dissociation or intoxication makes self-protection impossible.

Medication provides indirect protection by improving clarity, impulse control, and emotional stability. The young adult who is sleeping well, whose mood is stable, and whose thinking is clear is better equipped to recognize danger and extract themselves from harmful situations.

Clinicians should speak gently but directly about this dimension of treatment. One might say: "Stability helps protect you in situations where not everyone has your safety at heart." This is harm reduction, not moralizing. The clinician who avoids this topic out of discomfort fails to address a significant source of potential harm.

Stigma and Self-Stigma

For young adults, stigma is deeply personal and intersects with core developmental concerns. They fear being seen as broken or defective. They worry about romantic rejection if partners learn of their psychiatric history. They are concerned about career implications in competitive professional environments. They feel pressure to appear self-sufficient at precisely the developmental moment when self-sufficiency is the expected achievement.

Reframing medication in relation to identity can help. The clinician might say: "Medication doesn't change who you are. It protects who you are so that illness doesn't obscure the person you're becoming."

In this frame, taking medication becomes an act of self-respect rather than an admission of inadequacy.

VIII. Clinical Illustrations

A Long-Acting Injectable That Preserved a Semester

A nineteen-year-old college first-year student with emerging bipolar disorder cycled into mania every final exam period. The combination of sleep deprivation, academic pressure, and disrupted routine reliably destabilized her. Oral medication adherence crashed each time her schedule became chaotic—precisely when she needed stability most.

After her second hospitalization, she agreed to a long-acting injectable. The next semester, she passed all her courses—not because symptoms disappeared entirely, but because the ground beneath her stopped shifting. She could manage moderate symptoms; she could not manage the complete destabilization that oral medication non-adherence had repeatedly caused.

Cannabis, Chaos, and a Return to Clarity

A twenty-two-year-old man with a family history of bipolar disorder developed paranoia and panic after heavy cannabis use. He believed medication had failed him because symptoms worsened even while he was supposedly taking a mood stabilizer. What he did not initially recognize was that symptoms worsened when he stopped sleeping—and he stopped sleeping because of cannabis.

Psychoeducation about cannabis effects, combined with a structured mood stabilizer regimen and attention to sleep, allowed him to return to school and rebuild a sense of self he thought he had lost. He did not entirely stop cannabis use, but he reduced it substantially and became able to recognize when use was destabilizing him.

Exploitation in the Midst of Instability

A twenty-year-old woman with untreated mood disorder found herself repeatedly in coercive sexual situations she felt unable to escape. Sleep deprivation, alcohol use, and emotional volatility amplified her vulnerability. She described feeling as if she were watching herself make decisions she knew were dangerous, unable to intervene on her own behalf.

Stabilizing her mood and sleep dramatically altered her relationships and her ability to protect herself. She began recognizing predatory behavior earlier. She found herself able to leave situations that previously would have trapped her. Medication became part of her safety plan, restoring a sense of dignity and agency she feared she would never regain.

IX. Medicine and the Meaning

Young adults often worry that medication will alter their identity —that they will become someone different, someone less authentic, someone dependent on pills to be themselves.

The wiser question, which the clinician can help the young adult consider, is this: What parts of yourself do you want medication to protect so that you can become who you are meant to be?

Psychiatric illness, untreated, does not preserve authenticity. It obscures it. Depression flattens the personality. Mania distorts judgment and damages relationships. Anxiety constricts life into ever-smaller circles. Psychosis fragments the self. These are not authentic expressions of identity; they are illness imposing itself upon identity.

Medication, when it works, does not create a false self. It protects the emerging self from the distortions that illness would impose. It preserves possibility rather than diminishing it.

·　·　·

X. Closing Reflection

Young adulthood is not simply the end of adolescence; it is the beginning of authorship. The young adult is writing the first chapters of a life story that will continue for decades. Psychopharmacology in this period is a partnership in becoming.

Practiced with developmental sensitivity and deep respect for autonomy, medication becomes a stabilizing force when everything else is in motion. It serves as protection against derailment when illness threatens to push the young adult off course. It provides a foundation for growth by establishing the stability upon which development can proceed. It safeguards dignity and safety during a vulnerable period. It becomes a companion to the unfolding of a life story rather than an intrusion upon it.

When administered with wisdom, medication does not limit freedom, it creates it. The young adult who is stable can make choices; the one who is destabilized is driven by symptoms. The young adult who is protected can take risks; the one who is unprotected is merely reckless. The young adult who has pharmacological support can focus on becoming; the one without it is too often consumed by merely surviving.

This is the promise of psychopharmacology in young adulthood: not the replacement of the self, but the protection of the self during the threshold years when the foundations of life are being laid.

∼

7

PSYCHOPHARMACOLOGY IN MIDDLE ADULTHOOD

M iddle adulthood is often imagined as the era of steadiness: the time when identities have formed, careers have taken shape, relationships have matured, and life appears—at least from the outside—to have found a stable rhythm. Yet for many, this stage is not defined by stability at all, but by accumulated pressure, quiet suffering, and the gradual unraveling of coping mechanisms that once seemed sufficient.

This chapter explores the complexities of psychopharmacology in middle-aged adults, whose internal lives may be shaped by decades of emotional adaptation, unspoken burdens, and the friction between who they hoped to become and who life has required them to be.

Middle age is both a reckoning and an awakening.

I. THE DEVELOPMENTAL Landscape of Middle Adulthood
Middle adulthood, spanning approximately ages thirty-five to

sixty, is not a plateau—it is a landscape of multiple, often competing demands. Adults in this stage may find themselves raising children while simultaneously caring for aging parents, caught between generations that both require attention and energy. Careers that once felt like sources of identity and accomplishment may now generate increasing stress, whether from external pressures or internal questioning. Chronic illness often emerges or worsens during this period, adding physical burden to emotional strain. Relationships may be tested by divorce, loss, or the quieter erosion of connection that accumulates over years. Financial responsibilities frequently feel heavier than ever before, as the costs of children's education, aging parents' care, and retirement preparation converge. Traumas that were successfully buried for decades may resurface under the weight of accumulated stress. And for many, this is the period when meaning crises emerge—the unsettling question of whether this is truly the life they intended to live.

Symptoms in this stage often emerge gradually rather than dramatically, making them easy to normalize or dismiss. Worsening anxiety is mistaken for ordinary stress. Creeping depression is dismissed as burnout, an occupational hazard rather than a treatable illness. Mood instability is often seen as irritability or a challenging personality trait; while emerging bipolar disorder may be mistaken for a character trait instead of a medical condition. Cognitive fog is attributed to normal aging. Sleep disturbances are accepted as inevitable features of middle life.

These misinterpretations delay treatment and deepen suffering. The clinician who recognizes these patterns can intervene before years of additional deterioration occur.

II. The Complexity of Diagnosis in Midlife

Middle-aged adults have lived long enough to develop compensatory patterns that mask the true nature of their illness. Unlike younger patients whose symptoms may present more nakedly, those in midlife have often constructed elaborate adaptations that obscure what lies beneath.

Diagnostic challenges abound in this population. Symptoms may be camouflaged by coping strategies developed over decades. Comorbid medical conditions—thyroid disease, chronic pain, perimenopause, and menopause—create overlapping presentations that confuse the clinical picture. Long-term substance use may obscure mood patterns, making it difficult to determine what is primary and what is secondary. Traumas historically buried may become newly exposed by current stressors, producing symptoms that appear to emerge from nowhere. Personality adaptations can be misinterpreted as primary disorders, resulting in character-based diagnoses instead of appropriate treatment of the syndrome. Sleep disorders may mimic psychiatric symptoms so closely that the underlying cause is missed.

The clinician must untangle decades of narrative to understand what a symptom is, what is adaptation, and what is exhaustion. This requires patience, curiosity, and a willingness to revise initial impressions as the story unfolds.

Middle-aged adults often describe their suffering in terms of function rather than feeling. They report being unable to focus like they used to, or being irritable with their children, or losing patience at work. They say they do not feel like themselves anymore. Their emotional vocabulary may be muted, constrained by years of suppression or by cultural expectations that discourage emotional expression. Yet their distress, though understated, may be profound.

. . .

III. Medication in Midlife: A Different Meaning

In this stage of life, medication carries meanings distinct from those it holds in youth. The developmental context shapes how treatment is received and understood.

For some middle-aged adults, medication symbolizes failure. They believed they should have figured out how to manage by now. They expected that by this point in life, they would have mastered themselves sufficiently to need no external support. The prescription feels like an admission that decades of effort were insufficient.

For others, medication represents a last resort after years of silent endurance. They have been holding it together for so long, managing through sheer determination, and the need for medication signals that this approach has finally reached its limits.

For many, medication is experienced as acceptance— a recognition that something must change and that they cannot accomplish this change alone anymore. This acceptance, though it may be accompanied by grief, can also be the beginning of genuine recovery.

Middle-aged adults often struggle with shame rather than stigma. The distinction matters. Stigma is external—the fear of others' judgment. Shame is internal; the judgment they level against themselves for needing help after decades of self-reliance. This shame may be more difficult to address than external stigma because it operates silently within the patient's own mind.

The clinician's role is to gently challenge this shame, to help the patient recognize that reaching for help at this point is an act of wisdom rather than weakness. One might say something like: "You've carried so much for so long. Reaching for help now reflects how much you've already done, not how little."

IV. Medication Strategy in Middle Adulthood

Medication decisions in middle adulthood must account for the particular circumstances of this developmental stage. Several considerations shape pharmacologic choices.

Metabolic changes are becoming increasingly relevant. Weight gain, insulin resistance, and cardiovascular risk must be monitored carefully, and medications with significant metabolic effects may require either avoidance or close surveillance. The patient who could tolerate a particular medication in their twenties may experience different effects in their fifties.

Sleep restoration often emerges as a primary treatment target. Sleep is frequently the first system to break under chronic stress, and its restoration can be the first lever of recovery. Addressing sleep may produce improvements that extend far beyond nighttime hours.

Interactions with medical conditions shape pharmacologic choices in ways that may not have been relevant earlier in life. Hypertension, diabetes, autoimmune illness, perimenopause and menopause, and chronic pain all influence which medications are appropriate and which should be avoided. The clinician must coordinate with other providers and maintain awareness of the patient's full medical picture.

Substance use patterns require direct attention. Alcohol and cannabis are commonly used for self-soothing in this population, yet both can worsen mood, anxiety, and sleep. The patient may not initially recognize these connections, and the clinician must address them without judgment but with clarity.

Hidden bipolarity often emerges in this period. Late-diagnosed bipolar disorder frequently surfaces after years of being mislabeled as depression, anxiety, or irritability. The patient may have received multiple antidepressant trials that produced mixed results—initial improvement followed by agitation, or partial response followed by destabilization. A careful longitudinal history may reveal patterns that point toward a bipolar spectrum condition.

Emotional burnout may cause long-term coping mechanisms to collapse, requiring new medication strategies. This might include mood stabilizers, augmentation of existing medications, or a fundamental revisiting of old diagnoses that no longer seem adequate to explain the clinical picture.

V. The Turning Point: When Life Can No Longer Absorb the Symptoms

Middle-aged adults often seek treatment at a breaking point rather than during gradual decline. Something happens that makes the status quo impossible to maintain.

The collapse of a marriage may strip away the structure that had contained symptoms for years. Job loss or worsening work performance may threaten financial security and identity simultaneously. A child's mental health crisis may force parents to confront their own vulnerabilities while managing their child. Panic attacks may begin interrupting daily life in ways that cannot be hidden or ignored. The death or illness of a parent may remove an emotional anchor that had provided stability; or may trigger grief that overwhelms existing coping capacities. Fear of losing control of long-held responsibilities —of no longer being able to manage what one has always managed —may finally overcome resistance to seeking help.

At these moments, medication becomes not only treatment but stabilization for a life overloaded by responsibility. The patient needs to regain enough equilibrium to address the crisis, and medication may provide the foundation upon which other interventions can build.

. . .

VI. Clinical Illustrations

The Invisible Erosion

A forty-eight-year-old woman, mother of three and an admired professional, began waking at three in the morning overwhelmed with dread. She dismissed it as perimenopause, a hormonal nuisance that would eventually pass. Months went by. She withdrew from family meals, avoided friends who had once been sources of support, cried in the car before work while composing herself sufficiently to walk through the office door.

An SSRI briefly lifted her mood before agitation began to surface —restlessness, irritability, a driven quality that felt foreign to her. This was one of the hidden faces of bipolarity, activated by an antidepressant in a patient whose underlying mood disorder had never been recognized. When a mood stabilizer replaced the antidepressant, she finally felt present again. "I didn't realize how far I'd drifted from myself," she said. "I thought I was just tired."

The Light That Never Shut Off

A forty-two-year-old engineer was known at work for unmatched productivity and sudden waves of irritability that colleagues had learned to avoid. He believed this was simply his personality- high-energy, intense, occasionally difficult. He had always been this way, or at least he had been this way for as long as he could remember.

But when his marriage faltered under the strain of his volatility, he sought help for what he called "anger issues." His narrative, explored carefully over several sessions, revealed mixed-state bipolar symptoms- the combination of depressive cognition and manic energy that produces a particularly corrosive internal experience. A mood stabilizer quieted the internal engine that had been running at full throttle for decades. "I didn't know there was another way to live," he said. "I thought everyone felt like this inside."

The Weight of Two Generations

A fifty-five-year-old man caring for both his cognitively declining mother and his struggling adult son developed a deep depression. He assumed it was the burden of caregiving—a natural, perhaps inevitable response to impossible circumstances. Anyone would feel this way, he told himself.

But depression hollowed him out in ways that exceeded situational sadness. He lost the capacity to experience solace even in moments that should have provided it. Hope became inaccessible. He functioned, but only through mechanical effort that drained him further each day.

Medication lifted the haze enough for him to recognize that he had carried two generations on his back without rest, without acknowledgment, without anyone asking whether he himself was surviving. Treatment restored not only his functioning but his sense of worth-his recognition that he too deserved care, not only the capacity to provide it.

The Perfect Caregiver Who Forgot Herself

A fifty-two-year-old hospital administrator cared for everyone around her-her father with dementia, her daughter recovering from an eating disorder, her husband who traveled constantly for work and was emotionally absent even when present. She insisted she had no time to be the one who needed help. There was always someone whose needs were more pressing than her own.

But nightly wine escalated from one glass to three. Sleep crumbled into fragments. Agitation grew until she found herself snapping at colleagues who had done nothing wrong. An antidepressant prescribed by her internist worsened the irritability, revealing an underlying bipolar spectrum condition that the antidepressant had activated. A mood stabilizer quieted the storm that had been building for years.

"Why didn't anyone ever ask if I was okay?" she whispered during a session. The answer, of course, was that she had never allowed the question to be asked—had never presented herself as someone who might need asking.

The Executive Who Could No Longer Outrun His Mind

A forty-five-year-old executive, powered for decades by adrenaline and ambition, arrived in the office terrified after driving two hours on the highway with no memory of the route. He had arrived at his destination safely, but the missing time frightened him in a way nothing had before.

Panic and exhaustion had eroded his capacity to function, though he had hidden this erosion behind the competence that long practice had made automatic. He resisted medication, insisting he had always coped alone, that he did not need chemical assistance, that he should be able to manage this as he had managed everything else.

Finally, he admitted what he had never said aloud: "I've been white knuckling my life for twenty years." A combination of an SSRI and a low-dose beta-blocker gave him room to breathe—and, for the first time in decades, permission to rest.

Trauma That Waited Decades to Speak

A fifty-eight-year-old woman presented with what she called "late-life anxiety"—chest tightness, hypervigilance, intrusive memories that seemed to come from nowhere. She was puzzled by these symptoms, which had no obvious precipitant in her current circumstances.

Only later, as trust developed, did she reveal a history of childhood violence that had been buried for decades. She had survived by sealing those memories away, and the seal had held for most of her adult life. But the death of her mother—her last emotional anchor to the family system where the violence had occurred—unlocked memories that had been waiting behind a door she had believed was permanently closed.

Medication softened the acute symptoms enough to make trauma therapy possible. The therapy could not have proceeded without the stabilization that medication provided, and the medication alone would not have addressed what needed to be addressed. "I didn't know healing was still available to me," she said. "I thought it was too late."

The Collapsing Bridge Between Body and Mind

A fifty-year-old man with diabetes and hypertension repeatedly visited the emergency room with chest pain. Each time, cardiac evaluations were normal. His cardiologist was reassuring but increasingly puzzled.

His panic disorder, long unrecognized, was carving deep grooves into his body. The physical symptoms were real—the chest pain, the shortness of breath, the racing heart—but they originated in anxiety rather than cardiac disease. Yet the anxiety itself worsened his medical conditions: stress elevated his blood pressure, disrupted his sleep, and made diabetes management more difficult.

Medication restored his sleep and reduced the baseline anxiety that had been generating his symptoms. His blood pressure improved. His diabetes became easier to control. "I thought it was my heart," he reflected. "I didn't realize it was my life."

VII. The Soul of Treatment in Midlife

Middle-aged adults often need more than symptom relief. They arrive having survived, but survival is not the same as living. The work of treatment extends beyond pharmacology into domains that medication cannot directly address but help make accessible.

These patients need their meaning restored—a sense that their lives matter, that their efforts have purpose, that the years ahead hold something worth anticipating. They need dignity renewed—

the recognition that needing help does not diminish their worth. They need relationships repaired, or at least the capacity to attempt repair. They need long-held burdens acknowledged, often for the first time. They need permission to rest after decades of relentless effort. They need permission to ask for help without shame. They need permission to reclaim themselves after years spent serving others' needs.

Medication becomes one strand in a larger fabric of healing. It creates the stability that makes other work possible. It lifts the fog enough for clarity to emerge. It quiets the inner noise, enough for reflection to occur.

The work is not only to treat illness, but to help the person re-enter their own life after years spent simply surviving it.

VIII. Closing Reflection

Middle adulthood is not a time of decline—it is a time of transformation. The losses are real, but so are the possibilities.

Illness may surface during these years, but so does the wisdom to recognize it and seek help. Exhaustion may emerge, but so can the clarity that comes from finally acknowledging what has been carried too long.

This is when people finally say what they may never have said before: "I cannot keep living like this. I want something to change."

Psychopharmacology in this stage is a partnership in renewal. The clinician who approaches middle-aged patients with steadiness, empathy, and clinical precision offers something profound: not dependency, but freedom. Not the replacement of the self, but its restoration.

Medication in middle adulthood is an invitation—to stop merely surviving and to begin, perhaps for the first time in years, truly living.

8

PSYCHOPHARMACOLOGY
IN LATE LIFE

L ate life is often described as a period of decline, yet for many older adults it is a season of profound clarity, deepened perspective, and an unexpected expansion of emotional and spiritual life. It is a time shaped by accumulated wisdom, but also by new vulnerabilities—medical, cognitive, relational, and existential. Psychopharmacology in this stage requires careful balance: we must treat illness without dulling the very capacities that make late life meaningful.

Older adults carry long histories. They bring to treatment decades of identity formation, relationships built and sometimes lost, coping patterns refined through experience, traumas endured, losses absorbed, triumphs earned, and habits deeply ingrained. Their psychiatric symptoms arise not in a vacuum but in the rich, often complex context of a lifetime.

Medication in late life, therefore, is more than symptom relief. It is an opportunity to restore dignity, preserve functioning, support autonomy, and reduce suffering at a time when resilience meets biological change.

I. THE LANDSCAPE of Late Life

Late life presents a clinical landscape fundamentally different from earlier developmental stages. Both physiology and psychology have been transformed by decades of living, and treatment must account for these changes.

The body in late life operates under different rules. Metabolism slows, altering how medications are absorbed, distributed, and eliminated. Renal and hepatic function decline, sometimes subtly and sometimes dramatically, affecting drug clearance in ways that demand adjusted dosing. Sensitivity to medications increases, meaning that doses well-tolerated in younger adults may produce significant effects—both therapeutic and adverse—in older patients. The risk of side effects and drug interactions rises, particularly given the polypharmacy that often accompanies multiple medical conditions. Sleep architecture changes, with less deep sleep and more fragmentation, making sleep disturbances both more common and more consequential. Pain and medical comorbidities accumulate, adding layers of complexity to every treatment decision.

The psychology of late life is equally transformed. Grief accumulates as losses mount—the deaths of spouses, siblings, friends, and sometimes children create a landscape marked by absence. Fear of dependency haunts many older adults, who dread becoming burdens to those they love. Existential questioning intensifies as the horizon of remaining life becomes visible; questions of meaning, legacy, and mortality move from abstraction to immediacy. Social circles shrink through death, disability, and geographic separation, leaving some older adults profoundly isolated. Autonomy becomes fragile, threatened by physical limitation, cognitive change, and the well-meaning but sometimes infantilizing behavior of family members and institutions. Yet alongside these vulnerabilities, wisdom deepens. Many older adults achieve clarity about what matters, a capacity for perspective, and an emotional equanimity that younger people rarely possess.

In treating older adults, the clinician must recognize that symptoms arise from a lifetime, not merely from the present moment. Depression that appears at seventy-eight may have roots in losses from decades earlier. The anxiety that emerges at eighty-two may represent the surfacing of fears long suppressed. Understanding the patient requires understanding the life.

II. Diagnostic Complexity in Late Life

Psychiatric symptoms in older adults frequently mimic, overlap with, or emerge from conditions that are not primarily psychiatric. The differential diagnosis in late life is broader and more treacherous than at any other developmental stage.

Cognitive decline may produce symptoms that resemble depression, and depression may produce cognitive symptoms that resemble dementia. This pseudodementia—cognitive impairment that resolves with treatment of the underlying mood disorder—represents one of the most important diagnostic distinctions in geriatric psychiatry, because mistaking depression for dementia denies the patient treatment that could restore function. Medical illness can produce psychiatric symptoms directly; hypothyroidism causes depression, hyperthyroidism produces anxiety, and urinary tract infections in older adults may present with confusion and behavioral change rather than the classic symptoms seen in younger patients. Medication side effects account for a substantial proportion of psychiatric symptoms in older adults, given the polypharmacy that accompanies multiple medical conditions; what appears to be new-onset depression or anxiety may resolve when an offending medication is identified and discontinued. Grief and bereavement, though normal responses to loss, may shade into major depression, and distinguishing between them requires clinical judgment and longitudinal observation. Sensory impairment-particularly hearing and vision loss-can produce isolation, paranoia, and depressive symptoms that respond to sensory correction rather than psychiatric medication. Social isolation itself is a risk factor for depression and cognitive decline, and its effects may be addressed through environmental intervention rather than pharmacology. Chronic pain alters mood, disrupts sleep, and produces a syndrome that overlaps substantially with depression.

In this context, depression may appear not as sadness but as apathy, withdrawal, memory complaints, and slowed thinking. The older adult who seems to have given up, who no longer initiates activities or conversation, who moves and speaks slowly, may be experiencing a treatable mood disorder rather than the inevitable decline of aging. Anxiety may present primarily through somatic channels— chest tightness, gastrointestinal distress, shortness of breath—rather than through the psychological experience of worry that younger patients describe. Bipolar disorder may manifest as irritability, agitation, or late-life mania triggered by medications such as corticosteroids or by medical illness affecting the brain.

Diagnosis in late life must be slow, relational, and rooted in history. The clinician cannot rely on a single interview to understand what is happening. Information from family members, review of medical records, and observation over time are essential to accurate diagnosis.

.   .   .

III. Philosophy of Medication in Late Life

Pharmacotherapy in older adults requires a distinct philosophy, one that integrates biological caution with existential sensitivity.

The familiar adage "start low, go slow" captures an essential truth: older adults often require lower starting doses and more gradual titration than younger patients. Beginning at one-third to one-half the typical adult dose allows the clinician to assess response and tolerability before committing to higher doses. Yet this principle must be balanced against the recognition that undertreating suffering in the name of caution itself is harmful. When illness is severe, timely intervention matters, and excessive conservatism may prolong suffering unnecessarily.

The goal of treatment is to address suffering, not to treat age itself. Old age is not a disease, and the presence of advanced years does not itself constitute an indication for treatment nor does it constitute a contraindication. The question is always whether the patient is suffering, whether that suffering is treatable, and whether treatment can be provided safely.

Cognition must be protected at all costs. The mental clarity that allows older adults to maintain relationships, make decisions, and engage meaningfully with life is precious and fragile. Medications that cloud thinking—those with anticholinergic effects, excessive sedation, or cognitive side effects—should be avoided when alternatives exist. A treatment that relieves anxiety but produces confusion has not served the patient well.

Sleep restoration is a high priority in late-life treatment, as disordered sleep contributes to cognitive impairment, mood disturbance, and physical decline. Yet sleep must be restored carefully, using approaches that improve sleep architecture without producing morning sedation, falls, or dependence. The goal is restorative sleep, not pharmacological unconsciousness.

Life context must be considered deeply. An older adult's living situation, support system, medical conditions, functional status, and personal values all shape what treatment means and what it can accomplish. A medication that requires complex dosing may be inappropriate for someone with mild cognitive impairment and no caregiver. A treatment that interferes with the activities that give life meaning—reading, conversation, and time with grandchildren—may be worse than the condition it addresses.

Medication in late life is both biological and existential care. It addresses neurotransmitters and receptor systems, but it also addresses the patient's capacity to live a life that feels worth living. Both dimensions must be held in mind.

IV. Depression in Late Life

Late-life depression often differs from depression earlier in life, both in its presentation and in many meanings, it carries for the patient.

Depression in older adults frequently holds unresolved losses— the deaths of loved ones, the loss of physical capacities, the end of roles that once defined identity. Guilt about burdening others may torment patients who have spent their lives caring for family and who now find themselves in need of care. Existential despair may emerge as the patient contemplates a future that seems to hold only further decline. Cognition may be slowed, producing the pseudodementia that mimics degenerative illness.

Medication remains effective in late-life depression, though the choice of agent requires attention to the physiological changes of aging. SSRIs such as sertraline and escitalopram are generally well-tolerated and carry relatively low risk of drug interactions; they represent reasonable first-line options for many patients. Sertraline's mild dopaminergic effect may provide subtle activating properties that benefit patients with prominent apathy or fatigue. Escitalopram's clean pharmacology minimizes interaction concerns. Mirtazapine may be particularly useful when depression is accompanied by poor appetite, weight loss, and insomnia, as its side effect profile—increased appetite and sedation—may serve therapeutic purposes in this context. The sedation typically diminishes at higher doses, which may guide titration strategy. SNRIs such as venlafaxine and duloxetine offer options when depression coexists with chronic pain, as the noradrenergic effects may provide analgesic benefit; blood pressure monitoring is appropriate with these agents, particularly venlafaxine. Mood stabilizers should be considered when history suggests hidden bipolarity, as antidepressant monotherapy may destabilize patients with unrecognized bipolar spectrum conditions.

The stakes of treatment are high. Untreated depression in older adults accelerates physical and cognitive decline, increases mortality from medical illness, and robs patients of the capacity to engage with whatever time remains. Treatment restores not only mood but life itself.

V. Anxiety in Late Life

Older adults often experience anxiety differently from younger patients. The psychological experience of worry and dread may be less prominent than the bodily experience of distress. Anxiety appears in the chest, the gut, the muscles—as tightness, pain, nausea, and restlessness. The patient may seek medical attention for these physical symptoms without recognizing their psychiatric origin.

Safer long-term treatment options for late-life anxiety include SSRIs and SNRIs, which address anxiety effectively and can be titrated carefully to minimize side effects. Buspirone offers an alternative without sedation or dependence, though its delayed onset of action—requiring several weeks to achieve full effect—and need for consistent twice- or three-times-daily dosing may limit its utility for some patients. Gabapentin may be helpful when anxiety coexists with pain or insomnia, though it requires renal dose adjustment and may cause sedation or cognitive effects in some patients. Supportive therapy and cognitive-behavioral approaches complement pharmacotherapy and may reduce the medication burden.

Benzodiazepines should generally be avoided for routine anxiety management in older adults. The risks—falls with potential hip fractures, confusion that may mimic dementia, physiological dependence that complicates discontinuation—typically outweigh the benefits for chronic use. Brief, time-limited use may occasionally be appropriate, but the default should be alternative approaches.

VI. Bipolar Disorder in Late Life

Bipolar illness does not disappear with age. Patients diagnosed decades earlier continue to require mood stabilization, and new-onset mania can emerge in late life, sometimes triggered by medications or medical illness affecting the brain.

Late-life mania may be subtle, presenting as irritability, insomnia, and agitation rather than the grandiose euphoria of younger patients. The clinician must maintain a high index of suspicion when older adults present with sleep disturbance and behavioral change, particularly if there is any history of mood episodes or if current symptoms emerge after starting a new medication.

Treatment relies on mood stabilizers, with modifications for the physiological realities of aging. Lithium remains effective and may confer neuroprotective benefits, but it requires careful dosing and monitoring given age-related changes in renal function. Age-related decline in renal function means that doses appropriate earlier in life may produce toxic levels later; starting doses should be low, often 150 to 300 milligrams daily, with gradual titration guided by serum levels. Renal function and thyroid function should be monitored regularly. Valproate represents an alternative, though it carries risks of sedation, tremor, and drug interactions through hepatic enzyme inhibition. Lamotrigine offers mood stabilization with a relatively favorable side effect profile in older adults, though its slow titration requirement—necessitated by the risk of serious rash—means it is not suitable when rapid mood stabilization is needed. Atypical antipsychotics may be necessary for acute episodes but require vigilance regarding metabolic effects and, in patients with dementia, cerebrovascular risks that have prompted regulatory warnings.

VII. Psychosis and Delirium

The emergence of psychotic symptoms in late life demands a comprehensive medical evaluation before psychiatric treatment is considered. What appears to be new-onset schizophrenia or psychotic depression may in fact represent delirium, a medical emergency with psychiatric manifestations.

Delirium presents with fluctuating attention, hallucinations (often visual), disorientation, and sudden confusion that develops over hours to days rather than the gradual onset of primary psychiatric illness. The underlying cause may be infection, medication toxicity, metabolic disturbance, or any of dozens of other medical conditions. Treatment requires identifying and addressing the underlying cause; antipsychotic medications may reduce agitation but do not substitute for medical intervention.

When true late-life psychosis is diagnosed—whether as part of depression, bipolar disorder, or a primary psychotic illness—treatment with low-dose atypical antipsychotics may be appropriate. Risperidone, olanzapine, quetiapine, and aripiprazole have all been used in older adults, each with distinct side effect profiles that should guide selection for individual patients. Risperidone carries relatively higher risk of extrapyramidal symptoms. Olanzapine produces metabolic effects and sedation. Quetiapine's sedation may be useful for sleep but can impair daytime functioning. Aripiprazole's activating properties may benefit some patients but produce restlessness in others. All atypical antipsychotics require monitoring for metabolic effects, and all carry the regulatory warnings regarding use in patients with dementia.

VIII. Clinical Illustrations

The Quiet Descent

A seventy-eight-year-old widower withdrew from life in the two years following his wife's death. He stopped attending the church where he had been a deacon for decades. He declined invitations from his adult children. He spent his days in a chair by the window, eating little, speaking less.

He believed this was what grief was supposed to feel like. He believed he was simply experiencing what any man would experience after fifty-three years of marriage ended in loss. He did not recognize that grief had given way to something else— that major depression had quietly overtaken him.

Medication combined with therapy gradually rekindled meaning. He could not bring his wife back, but he could reengage with the grandchildren who had been puzzled by his withdrawal. He could return to church, not as he had been, but as someone who had endured and was now present again. "I thought I was supposed to disappear too," he said. "I didn't know there was another option."

Mania at Seventy-Two

A retired professor of history, known for his measured demeanor and scholarly precision, became sleepless, irritable, and grandiose after a course of corticosteroids for a respiratory illness. He began calling former colleagues at inappropriate hours with elaborate plans for a book series. He spent money he had carefully saved. His wife, alarmed by behavior she had never witnessed in forty-five years of marriage, brought him for evaluation.

This was first-onset mania, triggered by medication in a brain made vulnerable by age. A mood stabilizer restored clarity. He was embarrassed by his behavior during the episode, but he was grateful to understand what had happened. "I thought I was finally having the ideas I should have had years ago," he reflected. "I didn't realize I had lost my mind."

The Anxiety That Became a Prison

An eighty-two-year-old woman who had lived independently and actively became progressively homebound over the course of a year. She stopped driving, then stopped walking to the mailbox, then stopped leaving her bedroom. She described overwhelming fear—of falling, of strangers, of something terrible happening if she ventured beyond her door.

A gentle trial of an SSRI, started at a low dose and increased gradually, freed her from her internal captivity. Within weeks she was walking outside again. Within months she was resuming activities she had abandoned. "I didn't know what had happened to me," she said. "I just knew the world had become terrifying. And then it wasn't anymore."

The Misdiagnosed Dementia

A sixty-nine-year-old man was referred by his primary care physician for evaluation of cognitive decline. He had been forgetting appointments, losing track of conversations, struggling to complete tasks that had once been routine. His wife feared Alzheimer's disease.

Careful evaluation revealed severe depression with prominent cognitive symptoms. He had withdrawn from activities, slept poorly, and lost interest in the projects that had defined his retirement. Treatment of the depression—not the presumed dementia—restored his memory and his identity. "I thought I was losing myself," he said. "I didn't know I was sick in a way that could be fixed."

IX. Insomnia in Late Life

Sleep disturbance is among the most common complaints in older adults and among the most consequential. Poor sleep impairs cognition, worsens mood, increases risk for falls, and diminishes quality of life. Yet treating insomnia in this population requires particular care, as many traditional sleep aids carry unacceptable risks.

The first step in addressing late-life insomnia is identifying contributing factors. Pain, untreated depression or anxiety, medications with stimulating effects, sleep apnea, restless legs syndrome, and poor sleep hygiene all contribute to sleep disturbance and should be addressed before or alongside pharmacotherapy. Environmental factors—noise, light, an uncomfortable bed, a sleeping partner who snores—deserve attention.

When medication is needed, options that avoid the risks of benzodiazepines and traditional sedative-hypnotics are preferred. Melatonin may help regulate circadian rhythm with minimal side effects, though evidence for efficacy is modest and highly variable among individuals. Low-dose doxepin, a tricyclic antidepressant used at doses of three to six milligrams—far below those for depression—is FDA-approved for sleep maintenance insomnia in older adults and lacks the anticholinergic effects seen at antidepressant doses. Mirtazapine, when depression coexists with insomnia, can address both problems with a single medication, though weight gain may be a concern for some patients. Trazodone is commonly used for sleep, though orthostatic hypotension and next-day sedation require attention; starting doses should be low, typically twenty-five to fifty milligrams.

Benzodiazepines and non-benzodiazepine hypnotics such as zolpidem carry risks of falls, confusion, complex sleep behaviors, and dependence that generally make them poor choices for older adults. When used at all, they should be prescribed at the lowest effective dose for the shortest possible duration.

X. MEDICATIONS IN LATE LIFE: Principles, Preferences, and Precautions

The pharmacological treatment of older adults requires attention to principles that differ substantially from those guiding treatment earlier in life. Understanding these principles, recognizing which medications carry elevated risk, and knowing which agents are preferred for specific conditions together form the foundation of safe and effective prescribing in this population.

Dose Principles

The aging body handles medications differently than the younger body, and dosing must be adjusted accordingly. Starting low means beginning most psychiatric medications at one-third to one-half the dose that would be used in a healthy middle-aged adult. This conservative initiation allows the clinician to observe how the individual patient responds before committing to higher doses that may produce adverse effects. Going slow means extending the interval between dose increases, titrating over weeks rather than days, and resisting the pressure to escalate rapidly when improvement is not immediate. The older adult's response to medication often unfolds more gradually than the younger patients, and patience is rewarded with better tolerability.

Close monitoring encompasses multiple domains that may not require attention in younger patients. Laboratory values must be followed, particularly renal function for medications cleared by the kidneys and hepatic function for those metabolized by the liver. Vital signs deserve attention, as orthostatic hypotension from psychotropic medications can produce falls with devastating consequences. Cognition should be assessed at each visit because subtle confusion or slowed thinking may represent medication effect rather than disease progression. Fall risk must be evaluated, as sedation, dizziness, and impaired coordination from psychiatric medications contribute to fractures that can end independence or life itself.

Adjustment for organ function is not optional but essential. Renal clearance declines with age even when serum creatinine appears normal, because reduced muscle mass produces less creatinine to be cleared. Estimated glomerular filtration rate provides a more accurate assessment of renal function and should guide dosing of renally cleared medications such as lithium and gabapentin. Hepatic metabolism also slows, affecting medications processed through the cytochrome P450 system. The starting dose appropriate for a sixty-year-old with normal organ function may be excessive for an eighty-year-old with age-related decline in renal and hepatic capacity.

Avoiding sedation protects both cognition and mobility. Medications that produce drowsiness, mental clouding, or slowed reflexes impair the older adult's ability to think clearly, engage in meaningful activity, and move safely. A medication that controls anxiety but leaves the patient too foggy to read or converse has not served its purpose. The clinician must weigh the benefits of symptom control

against the costs of sedation and choose agents and doses that optimize the balance.

High-Risk Medications

Certain medication classes carry risks in older adults that generally outweigh their benefits, and clinicians should approach them
with caution or avoid them altogether.

Benzodiazepines represent one of the most significant sources of
iatrogenic harm in geriatric psychiatry. Their risks include falls,
which in older adults frequently result in hip fractures that carry
substantial morbidity and mortality. Cognitive impairment from
benzodiazepines may mimic dementia, leading to misdiagnosis and
inappropriate treatment. Physiological dependence develops readily,
and discontinuation after chronic use produces withdrawal symptoms that may include seizures. The half-lives of many benzodiazepines are prolonged in older adults, leading to accumulation and
toxicity even at doses that would be safe in younger patients.

Anticholinergic medications pose serious risks to the aging brain.
Cognitive decline, including both acute confusion and acceleration of
underlying dementing processes, represents the most concerning
effect. Peripheral anticholinergic effects include constipation, which
can progress to impaction and obstruction, and urinary retention,
which may precipitate infection or require catheterization. Many
medications have anticholinergic properties that are not immediately
obvious from their primary indication—certain antihistamines, anti-
spasmodics, and older antidepressants carry substantial anticholinergic burden. The cumulative anticholinergic load from multiple
medications may produce effects that no single agent would cause
alone.

Tricyclic antidepressants, once mainstays of depression treatment, have been largely supplanted by newer agents with more favorable safety profiles in older adults. Cardiac effects, including

prolongation of the QT interval and increased risk of arrhythmia, are particularly concerning in a population with high rates of cardiovascular disease. Orthostatic hypotension contributes to falls. Anticholinergic effects, prominent with many tricyclics, produce the cognitive and peripheral risks described above. Sedation impairs functioning and mobility. While tricyclics remain appropriate in selected situations, they are no longer first-line agents for most older adults with depression.

Sedating antipsychotics carry risks that extend beyond drowsiness. In patients with dementia, antipsychotics have been associated with increased risk of cerebrovascular events and mortality, leading to regulatory warnings that should inform prescribing decisions. Metabolic effects, including weight gain and glucose dysregulation, compound the medical burden in a population already managing multiple chronic conditions. Movement disorders, including tardive dyskinesia, may emerge and persist even after the medication is discontinued.

Diphenhydramine, available over the counter and often used for sleep, is particularly problematic in older adults. Its anticholinergic effects produce confusion, dry mouth, urinary retention, and constipation. Paradoxical agitation may occur. The medication's presence in many combination products means that patients may be exposed without realizing it. Clinicians should specifically ask about diphenhydramine use and educate patients about its risks.

The Perils of Polypharmacy

The accumulation of multiple medications represents one of the most significant safety concerns in late-life pharmacotherapy. Polypharmacy—typically defined as the concurrent use of five or more medications, though some definitions use higher thresholds— is nearly universal in older adults with chronic medical conditions, and its risks extend far beyond the additive side effects of individual agents.

Drug-drug interactions multiply with each medication added. Some interactions are pharmacokinetics, involving competition for metabolic enzymes or transport proteins that alter the levels of one or both medications. A patient stable on a medication for years may develop toxicity when a new agent is added that inhibits its metabolism. Other interactions are pharmacodynamic, involving additive or synergistic effects on the same physiological systems. Multiple medications with anticholinergic properties may produce cognitive impairment that no single agent would cause alone. Combinations of medications that lower blood pressure or prolong the QT interval may produce orthostatic hypotension or arrhythmia that would not occur with any single medication.

Adherence becomes increasingly difficult as regimens grow more complex. Medications taken at different times, with different instructions regarding food, with different frequencies, and from different prescribers create cognitive demands that may exceed what the patient can manage, particularly if any cognitive impairment is present. Non-adherence that results from complexity is not willful but practical, and simplifying regimens improves adherence more effectively than exhortation.

The prescribing cascade compounds polypharmacy when side effects of one medication are treated with another medication rather than recognized and addressed. The patient who develops ankle swelling from amlodipine receives furosemide; the furosemide produces urinary urgency that is treated with oxybutynin; the oxybutynin produces constipation treated with a laxative and confusion that may be mistaken for dementia. Each medication produces effects that generate additional prescriptions, and the patient accumulates a regimen that no single clinician would have designed.

Regular medication reconciliation is essential and potentially life-saving. At every visit, the clinician should review all medications the patient is taking—prescribed, over the counter, and supplemental-and ask why each one is being used. Medications initiated for conditions that have been resolved, medications that duplicate the effects of other agents, medications producing side effects that impair quality of life, and medications whose risks now outweigh their benefits should be identified for discontinuation or substitution. Deprescribing—the systematic process of reducing medication burden—has emerged as a discipline in its own right, recognizing that stopping medications may be as important as starting them.

Communication among prescribers is often inadequate, with each specialist managing their own domain without awareness of what others have prescribed. The primary care clinician may not know about the antipsychotic the psychiatrist added; the psychiatrist may not know about the benzodiazepine the primary care clinician continued from a hospitalization. A single clinician or pharmacist should serve as the coordinator of the medication regimen, maintaining a comprehensive list and evaluating each new prescription in the context of the whole.

The patient and family are essential partners in managing polypharmacy. They should be encouraged to maintain their own medication list, to bring all medications to appointments, and to question new prescriptions. They should understand that more medications are not necessarily better and that simplification of the regimen is a worthy goal. When cognitive impairment limits the patient's ability to participate in this process, a caregiver should assume the role.

XI. Closing Reflection

Late life is not merely decline—it is integration, reflection, possibility, and often profound growth. The older adult has accumulated a lifetime of experience, loss, and wisdom. The clinician who dismisses this stage as simply a period of deterioration misses both the suffering that can be treated and the capacities that must be preserved.

Psychopharmacology in late life must be practiced with humility and reverence. The clinician holds responsibility not only for treating symptoms but for protecting the patient's ability to live whatever time remains with clarity, dignity, and meaning.

We restore functioning that illness has taken. We protect cognition that makes relationship and reflection possible. We reduce suffering that need not be endured. We honor the life lived—and we safeguard the life that remains.

∼

PART III

9

MEN'S ISSUES

SILENCE, STOICISM, AND
THE COST OF ENDURANCE

M en often arrive in psychiatric care late—not because they suffer less, but because they suffer quietly. From an early age, many men are trained to endure rather than express, to function rather than feel, to provide rather than receive care. Emotional distress is frequently reframed as weakness, fatigue as failure, and vulnerability as something to be hidden or overridden.

Psychopharmacology with men therefore requires more than diagnostic accuracy. It requires sensitivity to silence, respect for stoicism, and an understanding of the deep cultural, biological, and psychological forces that shape how men experience illness and seek —or avoid—help.

When men finally present for treatment, they are often already depleted. Medication becomes not only a tool for symptom relief, but an intervention that can interrupt years of unspoken suffering and prevent irreversible losses.

. . .

I. THE MALE Experience of Distress

Men are less likely to articulate sadness or fear. Instead, distress often appears through channels that obscure its emotional origins. Irritability and anger may dominate the clinical picture, masking the despair that drives them. Emotional withdrawal creates distance from relationships and from the feelings themselves. Risk-taking behaviors —driving too fast, drinking too much, seeking danger—may represent attempts to feel something, to escape numbness, or to court an ending that cannot be spoken aloud. Substance use provides temporary relief from internal states that have no other outlet. Workaholism transforms suffering into productivity, allowing the man to outrun his pain until exhaustion forces a reckoning. Somatic complaints—headaches, back pain, fatigue, gastrointestinal distress —give bodily form to emotional experiences that have no psychological language. And sometimes, after years of overextension, there is sudden functional collapse: the man who never missed a day of work cannot get out of bed; the provider who held everything together falls apart without warning.

Many men seek help only when symptoms threaten their ability to work, provide, or maintain control. Emotional pain is tolerated, sometimes for decades. Functional failure is not. The man who would never consult a psychiatrist for sadness may present urgently when he can no longer perform his job. The man who dismissed anxiety as something to push through may seek help when panic attacks threaten his capacity to drive or to appear competent before colleagues.

This pattern shapes how men present, what they disclose, and what remains hidden. The clinician who listens only for the classic presentations of psychiatric illness will miss much of what men experience. The clinician who understands that distress speaks through many languages—anger, silence, action, the body, the bottle—will recognize suffering that has learned to disguise itself.

II. Diagnostic Patterns in Men
Depression

Depression is underdiagnosed in men and often misinterpreted. The cultural expectation that men should not feel or express sadness leads many men to experience depression through alternative channels and leads many clinicians to miss the diagnosis when it presents atypically.

Men with depression may present with anger rather than sadness. The irritability that emerges may be directed at family members, coworkers, or strangers; it may produce conflict, isolation, and the erosion of relationships that might otherwise provide support. Emotional numbing replaces the tearfulness that clinicians expect; the man describes feeling nothing rather than feeling sad, and this absence of feeling may be mistaken for absence of illness. Loss of motivation manifests as difficulty initiating tasks, abandoning hobbies and interests, and withdrawal from activities that once provided meaning—yet without the expressed hopelessness that would signal depression to an observer. Increased substance use may represent self-medication, an attempt to manage intolerable internal states through alcohol or drugs. Reckless behaviors-financial, sexual, physical-may reflect the impulsivity of depression or an unconscious movement toward self-destruction.

Most concerning, suicidal ideation in men often occurs without verbalized despair. The man who is planning to end his life may appear calm, even relieved, having made a decision that resolves his internal conflict. He may not report suicidal thoughts unless specifically asked, and even then, may minimize or deny them. Male suicide rates are significantly higher than female rates—in many countries, three to four times higher—underscoring the danger of missed or minimized depression. The man who appears to be coping may be dying.

Anxiety

Anxiety in men is often masked by control strategies. The man who experiences overwhelming fear may respond by tightening his grip on every aspect of life, becoming rigid, perfectionistic, and controlling in ways that create conflict but obscure the underlying terror. Avoidance may be subtle: the man stops accepting social invitations, finds reasons not to travel, gradually narrows his world without acknowledging why. Panic attack may present itself as chest pain, dizziness, shortness of breath, or fear of losing control; these physical symptoms prompt cardiac workups and emergency department visits while the psychiatric origin goes unrecognized. The man who presents to the emergency room convinced he is having a heart attack, whose cardiac enzymes are normal and whose ECG is unremarkable, may have panic disorder—and may resist this diagnosis as somehow less legitimate than a physical illness.

Bipolar Disorder

Bipolar disorder in men may present with externalizing behaviors that lead to misdiagnosis. Impulsivity, aggression, substance use, and reckless behavior during manic or hypomanic episodes may be attributed to character flaws, personality disorder, or conduct problems rather than recognized as symptoms of a mood disorder. The man with undiagnosed bipolar disorder may accumulate legal problems, failed relationships, and employment difficulties; he may be labeled as irresponsible, volatile, or antisocial; he may internalize these judgments and understand himself as fundamentally flawed rather than ill. Accurate diagnosis reframes years of struggle and opens the possibility of effective treatment.

Attention-Deficit/Hyperactivity Disorder

ADHD is often identified earlier in males than in females, as the hyperactive and impulsive presentations that predominate in boys draw attention in school settings. Yet the disorder does not disappear with childhood. Emotional dysregulation, executive dysfunction, difficulty with organization and follow-through, and problems with impulse control persist into adulthood, complicating mood disorders and contributing to substance use. The man whose childhood ADHD was treated may have discontinued medication in adolescence or young adulthood, only to find his symptoms reemerging as adult responsibilities exceed his executive capacity. The man whose ADHD was never diagnosed may have developed elaborate compensatory strategies that mask the underlying disorder while exacting enormous effort.

III. Masculinity, Identity, and the Meaning of Medication

For many men, the prospect of psychiatric medication challenges deeply held beliefs about self-sufficiency, strength, and identity. These beliefs are often unspoken but powerful, shaping the man's response to the very idea of treatment.

"I should handle this on my own." The man who has built his identity around self-reliance experiences the need for help as failure. He may have been taught, explicitly or implicitly, that real men solve their own problems, which asking for help is weakness, that depending on others—or on medication—represents a fundamental inadequacy. This belief system may have served him in some contexts, enabling perseverance through difficulty, but it becomes an obstacle when illness exceeds what willpower can manage.

"Needing help means I failed." The equation of help-seeking with failure transforms treatment into an admission of defeat. The man may delay seeking care for years, hoping that effort or time will resolve what only treatment can address. By the time he presents, he may be deeply ashamed—ashamed of his symptoms, ashamed of his inability to overcome them, ashamed of being in a psychiatrist's office at all.

"Medication will make me weak." The fear that psychiatric medication will alter personality, diminish drive, or create dependence may deter men from accepting treatment even when they acknowledge their suffering. This fear often reflects misunderstanding of how psychiatric medications work, but it also reflects a deeper concern about authenticity and autonomy: Will I still be me? Will I be able to function without it? Will I become someone I don't recognize?

These concerns deserve respect rather than dismissal. The clinician who brushes aside a man's hesitation about medication misses an opportunity to build alliance and may provoke the very resistance that leads to non-adherence or treatment dropout.

Reframing medication as restoring capacity rather than diminishing strength can shift the conversation. "This is not about changing who you are. It's about helping you function at your best." When framed as performance support, stability, or recovery of agency, medication becomes compatible with masculine identity rather than threatening to it. The man who would reject a "crutch" may accept a tool. The man who would refuse to be "fixed" may embrace being restored.

The language matters. Discussing how medication can help the man return to work, be present for his family, sleep through the night, or regain the energy and focus that illness has stolen speaks to values he already holds. Meeting him where he is—honoring his identity while addressing his illness—creates the conditions for engagement.

. . .

IV. Biological Considerations in Men

Testosterone and Mood

Testosterone levels decline gradually with age, and this decline may contribute to symptoms that overlap with psychiatric illness. Fatigue, irritability, low mood, reduced motivation, decreased libido, and difficulty concentrating may all accompany low testosterone. For some men, these symptoms respond to testosterone replacement; for others, they reflect mood disorder, medical illness, or lifestyle factors that testosterone will not address.

The relationship between testosterone and mood is complex and bidirectional. Low testosterone may contribute to depression, but depression itself can lower testosterone levels. Treating depression sometimes normalizes testosterone; replacing testosterone sometimes improves mood. Yet psychiatric symptoms should not be reflexively attributed to testosterone alone. A man with major depression requires treatment for depression, regardless of his testosterone level. A man with normal testosterone who receives replacement therapy for presumed deficiency will not benefit and may experience adverse effects.

When testosterone deficiency is suspected, laboratory evaluation can clarify the picture. When deficiency is confirmed and symptoms are consistent, replacement may be appropriate in collaboration with an endocrinologist or primary care physician experienced in hormone management. When psychiatric illness is present, it requires independent evaluation and treatment.

Sleep Apnea

Obstructive sleep apnea is highly prevalent in men and profoundly underdiagnosed. The disorder disrupts sleep architecture, produces oxygen desaturation, and prevents the restorative rest that maintains mood, cognition, and physical health. Men with untreated sleep apnea experience fatigue, irritability, difficulty concentrating, and depressed mood—symptoms that may prompt psychiatric referral while the underlying cause goes unaddressed.

Untreated sleep apnea worsens depression and anxiety, impairs cognitive function, and diminishes response to psychiatric medication. The man who has failed multiple antidepressant trials may have sleep apnea that prevents any medication from working optimally. Risk factors include obesity, large neck circumference, snoring, witnessed apneas, and daytime sleepiness, but the disorder can occur in men without obvious risk factors.

Screening for sleep apnea should be routine in men presenting with mood or cognitive symptoms. When clinical suspicion exists, polysomnography or home sleep testing can confirm the diagnosis. Treatment with continuous positive airway pressure or other interventions may produce improvements in mood and cognition that exceed what psychiatric medication alone can achieve.

Cardiovascular Risk

Men are at higher baseline risk for cardiovascular disease than premenopausal women, and this risk shapes medication selection. Psychiatric medications vary in their metabolic and cardiac effects; some promote weight gain, glucose dysregulation, and lipid abnormalities that compound cardiovascular risk, while others are relatively neutral or even favorable.

When treating men with cardiovascular risk factors—or men in whom such risk factors may develop—the clinician should prefer medications with favorable metabolic profiles when efficacy is comparable. Monitoring weight, blood pressure, fasting glucose, and lipid panels allows early detection of adverse metabolic trends. Collaboration with primary care ensures that cardiovascular risk is managed comprehensively rather than in isolation.

. . .

V. Substance Use: A Central Axis of Male Psychopathology

Men have higher rates of alcohol use disorder, stimulant misuse, cannabis dependence, and risk-taking behavior under intoxication than women. Substance use is woven through male psychopathology so pervasively that it cannot be addressed as a separate issue; it must be integrated into every aspect of assessment and treatment.

Substances are often used as emotional regulators. The man who cannot identify or express his feelings may discover that alcohol quiets anxiety, that stimulants lift depression, that cannabis numbs pain. What begins as self-medication becomes dependence; what began as a solution becomes a problem that compounds the original suffering.

Shame and cultural norms delay disclosure. The man who drinks heavily may minimize his consumption, fearing judgment or the implication that he cannot handle his liquor. The man who uses cocaine may conceal this entirely, aware that disclosure changes how he will be perceived. The clinician must create conditions in which honesty is possible— asking directly about substance use, normalizing the question, responding without judgment to whatever is disclosed.

Assessment of substance use must be specific and quantitative. Asking "Do you drink?" invites the answer "socially" from men who consume dangerous amounts. Asking "How many drinks in a typical week?" and "What's the most you've had in a single day in the past month?" yields actionable information. Similar specificity applies to other substances.

Treatment must integrate substance use into medication planning. Active heavy drinking complicates every psychiatric condition and undermines every psychiatric treatment. Stimulant misuse may contraindicate stimulant treatment for comorbid ADHD or may require carefully structured treatment with close monitoring. Cannabis use, often perceived as benign, can worsen anxiety, impair motivation, and destabilize mood in vulnerable individuals.

When substance use disorder is present, it requires treatment—not as a precondition for psychiatric care, but as an integral part of it. Medications for alcohol use disorder, such as naltrexone and acamprosate, may be combined with antidepressants or mood stabilizers. Integrated treatment that addresses both substance use and psychiatric illness produces better outcomes than sequential treatment of either condition alone.

VI. Trauma in Men: The Unspoken History

Men experience trauma at high rates, but this trauma often remains unspoken—sometimes for decades, sometimes forever. The cultural expectation that men should be invulnerable, combined with specific stigma around certain forms of victimization, creates barriers to disclosure that may never be overcome.

Childhood abuse—physical, emotional, and sexual—affects boys as well as girls, though boys may be less likely to disclose, less likely to be asked, and less likely to receive intervention. The abused boy becomes a man who carries his history silently, its effects evident in his relationships, his emotional life, and his psychiatric symptoms, but its origins hidden even from those who try to help him.

Violence exposure, whether as victim or witness, shapes development and leaves lasting effects. Boys growing up in violent homes or violent neighborhoods learn survival strategies that may become maladaptive in other contexts. The hypervigilance that protected him as a child becomes the anxiety that impairs him as an adult.

Combat trauma produces specific forms of injury in those who serve in military roles. The veteran may experience intrusive memories, hyperarousal, emotional numbing, and difficulty readjusting to civilian life. He may resist the label of PTSD, viewing it as weakness or as a repudiation of his service. He may disclose his combat experience but not his symptoms, or his symptoms but not their connection to what he witnessed and did.

Occupational trauma affects first responders, healthcare workers, and others exposed repeatedly to death, suffering, and threat. The cumulative burden of these exposures may exceed what any individual can process, producing symptoms that emerge years into a career.

Sexual trauma in men is vastly underreported. The man who was assaulted—whether in childhood, adolescence, or adulthood—may have told no one. He may experience shame so profoundly that disclosure feels impossible. He may not frame his experience as assault or abuse, lacking the language or the permission to name what happened. The clinician who assumes that trauma means combat or childhood physical abuse may miss the man whose suffering has entirely different origins.

Trauma in men frequently manifests as anger, emotional shutdown, or substance use rather than the fear and sadness that clinicians associate with PTSD. The man who presents with rage may be traumatized. The man who feels nothing may be traumatized. The man who drinks to blackout may be traumatized. Recognizing trauma requires looking beyond the presenting symptoms to the history that shaped them.

Medication addresses the biological dysregulation that trauma produces—the hyperarousal, sleep disruption, the mood instability — but medication alone is insufficient. Trauma-informed treatment requires an alliance in which the man feels safe enough to approach what he has avoided, language that neither minimizes nor sensationalizes his experience, and patience for a process that cannot be rushed. "You don't have to carry this alone" may be the most therapeutic statement the clinician can make.

VII. Clinical Illustrations

The Man Who Never Missed a Day

A fifty-two-year-old construction supervisor presented to the emergency department convinced he was having a heart attack. His chest was tight, his heart racing, his hands trembling. He had never been sick. He had never missed a day of work in thirty years. He had raised four children, buried his parents, supported his wife through cancer treatment, and never complained.

The cardiac workup was normal. And then normal again when he returned two weeks later with the same symptoms. And normal a third time, when he came back convinced that something had been missed.

What had been missed was severe anxiety and depression, masked by decades of endurance. He had never allowed himself to feel what he felt; he had only allowed himself to function. When functioning finally failed—when his body could no longer contain what his mind refused to acknowledge—it spoke the only language left to it: the language of physical crisis.

An SSRI restored sleep within weeks. The panic attacks subsided. The chest tightness eased. But more than symptoms resolved; something opened in him that had been closed for as long as he could remember. He began to speak about his father's death, about the fear he had carried during his wife's illness, about the loneliness of always being the strong one.

"I didn't know I was allowed to stop," he said quietly. "I didn't know anyone would catch me if I fell."

Anger as Depression

A thirty-eight-year-old man was referred by his employer for anger management after a confrontation with a coworker that nearly became physical. He arrived resentful, viewing the referral as punishment rather than help. He denied depression. He denied anxiety. He denied needing to be there at all.

What emerged over several sessions was profound depression that had worn the mask of anger for years. He was not an angry man; he was a despairing man whose despair had no acceptable form of expression. He was emotionally numb, going through the motions of life without feeling present for any of it. He was ashamed—of his failures, his inadequacies, his inability to be the man he thought he should be. The anger was not the problem; the anger was the only outlet for pain that had nowhere else to go.

Medication reduced irritability and emotional reactivity. What it uncovered was sadness that he had not allowed himself to feel since childhood. For the first time in his adult life, he cried in another person's presence. The anger had protected him from this vulnerability; releasing the anger meant feeling what lay beneath it. This was not easy. It was not quick. But it was the beginning of something he had never experienced: an authentic emotional life.

The Late Diagnosis

A forty-five-year-old entrepreneur had built three companies, lost two of them, and was working ninety-hour weeks to save the third. He described his life as a series of cycles: periods of extraordinary productivity, creativity, and confidence, followed by crashes in which he could barely function. He had always attributed this to the demands of entrepreneurship, to the natural rhythm of building and losing, to his own character.

What he described was bipolar II disorder, unrecognized for more than two decades. The hypomanic episodes had fueled his business ventures; the depressive episodes had nearly destroyed him. He had never sought help during the depressions, viewing them as personal weakness. He had never questioned the episodes of hypomania, experiencing them as his best self.

A mood stabilizer brought balance—not the artificial flattening he had feared, but a steadiness he had never known. The relentless internal pressure eased. He could work without being driven. He could rest without collapsing. He could make decisions based on judgment rather than the urgency of an altered brain state.

"I thought this was just who I was," he said. "I didn't know there was another way to live."

Trauma Without Words

A veteran in his early thirties presented with insomnia and irritability. He had served two deployments. He was not sleeping more than three or four hours a night, and his wife had moved to the guest room because he thrashed and shouted in his sleep. He was short-tempered with his children in ways that frightened him.

He denied fear. He denied nightmares—or rather, he said he didn't remember his dreams. He denied that his service had affected him. He was fine. He just needed something for sleep.

What emerged slowly, over months of treatment, was a trauma history he had never disclosed to anyone. He had witnessed things he could not erase from his memory. He had done things that violated his own moral code. He had lost friends in ways that made survival feel like betrayal. He carried all of this silently, believing that speaking it would be weakness, that a real soldier would handle it, that his suffering was less legitimate than that of those who had not come home.

Medication addressed the hyperarousal—prazosin reduced the nightmares; an SSRI eased the hair-trigger reactivity. He began to sleep. He began to feel less like a danger to his own family.

But the healing that mattered most began when he was told in simple words that he could hear them: "You don't have to carry this alone. What you're experiencing makes sense given what you went through. And there's no weakness in getting help— there's courage."

He wept in a way he had not allowed himself to weep since he was a child. The tears were not the end of treatment. They were the beginning.

VIII. Medication Approaches in Men

Pharmacological treatment in men requires the same diagnostic precision as in any population, but the approach must be tailored to the patterns of presentation, the biological considerations, and the psychological meanings that shape how men experience both illness and treatment.

Depression

SSRIs and SNRIs remain first-line treatments for depression in men, as in other populations. Sertraline, escitalopram, and fluoxetine are well-established options with extensive safety data. SNRIs such as venlafaxine and duloxetine may be particularly useful when depression is accompanied by chronic pain or when fatigue and low energy are prominent features. Bupropion, with its activating profile and absence of sexual side effects, may be preferred by men for whom sexual dysfunction would be intolerable or would lead to discontinuation. The man who stops his antidepressant because it impairs his sexual function is not being helped, regardless of its efficacy for mood.

When depression presents with irritability and anger, these symptoms should be monitored as treatment targets. Improvement in mood may manifest first as reduced reactivity, greater patience, and less interpersonal conflict before the man experiences or reports feeling better emotionally. Asking about these behavioral markers may reveal treatment response that the man would not spontaneously describe.

Suicidal ideation requires direct assessment in every man with depression. The question must be asked explicitly; it will not be volunteered. The man who appears to be coping may be actively planning his death. The man who denies depression may nonetheless be suicidal. Safety assessment and safety planning are essential components of treatment.

Anxiety

SSRIs are effective for anxiety disorders in men, though the initial activation that some patients experience may be particularly problematic for men who are already irritable or who interpret anxiety symptoms as loss of control. Starting at lower doses and titrating slowly can minimize this activation. Buspirone provides an alternative without sedation, sexual side effects, or the dependence potential of benzodiazepines; its delayed onset of action requires patient education about expectations. Cognitive-behavioral therapy, when accessible and acceptable to the patient, provides skills that may reduce reliance on medication and produce durable improvement.

Benzodiazepines carry particular risks in men with substance use histories. The man who has used alcohol to manage anxiety may readily transfer this pattern to benzodiazepines, developing dependence and requiring escalating doses. When benzodiazepines are used, they should be prescribed with clear limits, for defined indications, and with ongoing assessment of use patterns.

Bipolar Disorder

Mood stabilizers are the foundation of treatment for bipolar disorder in men, as in all populations. Lithium, valproate, and lamotrigine each have roles depending on the clinical picture, the phase of illness, and the patient's medical status. Lithium's demonstrated efficacy for suicidality makes it particularly important in a population at elevated suicide risk.

When bipolar disorder is presented primarily through external-izing behaviors—impulsivity, aggression, and substance use— the clinician must educate the patient about the nature of the disorder. The man who has understood himself as having a character flaw or a substance problem must come to understand that he has a brain-based illness that distorts judgment and drives behavior. This reframing is therapeutic in itself, relieving shame and creating the foundation for adherence to treatment.

ADHD

Stimulant medications remain the most effective treatment for ADHD in adults, including men whose childhood diagnoses have persisted or whose ADHD has been recognized only in adulthood. Methylphenidate and amphetamine formulations, particularly extended-release preparations, reduce symptoms and improve func-tioning for most patients. Atomoxetine and viloxazine provide non-stimulant alternatives when stimulants are contraindicated or not tolerated.

In men with histories of substance use disorder, stimulant prescribing requires careful consideration. Active addiction is gener-ally a contraindication to stimulant treatment, or at minimum requires highly structured prescribing with close monitoring. Stable recovery does not preclude stimulant use, but the decision should be made collaboratively, with attention to the patient's own assessment of risk and with safeguards in place. For some men, non-stimulant options are preferable regardless of efficacy differences, because the risks of stimulant diversion or misuse are too high.

Insomnia

Sleep disturbance in men often reflects underlying depression, anxiety, or substance use, and treating the primary condition may resolve the insomnia without specific sleep-focused intervention. When insomnia persists or is severe, treatment should generally avoid benzodiazepines and traditional hypnotics, which carry risks of dependence and next-day impairment.

Cognitive-behavioral therapy for insomnia, when available, provides durable improvement without medication. Trazodone at low doses, melatonin, and low-dose doxepin offer pharmacological options with more favorable risk profiles than benzodiazepines. For men with trauma-related nightmares, prazosin can reduce nightmare frequency and intensity, improve sleep quality, and reduce the dread of sleep that compounds insomnia.

Monitoring Considerations

Cardiovascular and metabolic monitoring is particularly important in men, given baseline risk profiles. Weight, blood pressure, fasting glucose, and lipid panels should be obtained at baseline and monitored regularly, with frequency determined by the patient's risk factors and the metabolic profile of prescribed medications.

Sexual function should be assessed, as sexual side effects are common with many psychiatric medications and may lead to non-adherence if not addressed. Men may not spontaneously report sexual dysfunction, whether from embarrassment or from uncertainty about whether it relates to medication. Direct inquiry normalizes the topic and opens the door to intervention—dose adjustment, medication switching, or adjunctive treatment as appropriate.

IX. Closing Reflection

For many men, the bravest act is not endurance but asking for help. The cultural training that equates strength with silence and self-sufficiency with worth creates barriers to care that cost lives. Men die by suicide at rates that dwarf those of women, not because they suffer more but because they suffer alone.

Psychopharmacology becomes a bridge—from silent suffering to restored agency, from isolation to engagement, from collapse to continuity. Medication does not diminish masculinity; it restores the capacity to live, work, connect, and endure without breaking.

The clinician who treats men must learn to hear what is not said, to see distress in its disguised forms, to create space for vulnerability without demanding it. The man who has never spoken his pain needs a listener who can tolerate silence while remaining present. The man who speaks only through anger needs a clinician who can hear the grief beneath. The man who has built his identity around strength needs a clinician who can redefine strength to include the courage of seeking help.

We do not ask men to become something other than who they are. We help them become who they are more fully—not diminished by illness, not imprisoned by silence, not destroyed by what they refuse to feel. Medication is one part of this work, but only one part. The larger work is relational, cultural, and ultimately human: the work of teaching men that they are allowed to suffer, allowed to speak, and allowed to heal.

∾

10

WOMEN'S ISSUES
THE BODY AS LANDSCAPE, THE MIND AS WITNESS

To treat women wisely in psychopharmacology is to understand that their bodies are not static vessels but shifting landscapes—shaped by hormones, seasons of life, cultural expectations, burdens carried silently, and strengths often unseen. A woman's psychology is lived through a body that changes in ways that men's do not: cyclically, rhythmically, biologically, socially, and symbolically.

Women encounter unique vulnerabilities and equally unique forms of resilience. Their suffering is often minimized, mislabeled, or attributed to personality rather than biology. Their requests for help may be softened, encoded, or framed apologetically. Yet when a woman suffers, her suffering radiates outward—touching children, partners, parents, communities—and when she heals, healing radiates outward as well.

Psychopharmacology with women requires attentiveness not only to diagnosis and dose, but to context, timing, relationships, biology, and the unspoken stories embedded in their lives. The clinician who treats women must learn to read what is not said, to understand symptoms in context, and to offer treatment that honors both the complexity of female biology and the weight of female experience.

I. THE FEMALE Body as a Changing Neurobiological Landscape

Women's psychiatric symptoms unfold within a dynamic hormonal environment that has no true parallel in men. From menarche to menopause and beyond, the female brain operates in constant dialogue with fluctuating levels of estrogen, progesterone, and other hormones that influence neurotransmitter systems, neural plasticity, stress reactivity, and cognitive function. Understanding this dialogue is essential to understanding how psychiatric illness presents, evolves, and responds to treatment in women.

The menstrual cycle creates a monthly rhythm of hormonal change that affects mood, anxiety, sleep, cognition, and energy. Estrogen rises during the follicular phase, peaks at ovulation, then falls as progesterone rises during the luteal phase; both hormones decline before menstruation. For many women, these fluctuations are experienced as subtle shifts in well-being—mild changes in energy or mood that are noticeable but not impairing. For others, particularly those with premenstrual dysphoric disorder, the luteal phase brings profound changes: severe irritability, depression, anxiety, and physical symptoms that impair functioning and relationships, then resolve with the onset of menstruation. The cyclical nature of these symptoms is diagnostic; the suffering is not merely "hormonal" in the dismissive sense but represents a genuine neurobiological vulnerability to hormonal change.

Pregnancy initiates a profound neuroendocrine reorganization. Rising levels of estrogen and progesterone, changes in the hypothalamic-pituitary-adrenal axis, and alterations in neurotransmitter systems create an internal environment unlike any other in a woman's life. For some women, pregnancy brings emotional stability and even remission of prior psychiatric symptoms. For others, it brings new-onset illness or exacerbation of existing conditions. The decision about whether to continue, modify, or discontinue psychiatric medication during pregnancy is among the most consequential a woman and her clinician will face—and it must be made with attention to risks that run in both directions.

The postpartum period represents an abrupt hormonal withdrawal superimposed on sleep deprivation, physical recovery, identity transformation, and the overwhelming demands of caring for a newborn. Estrogen and progesterone, which rose steadily throughout pregnancy, but plummets within hours of delivery. This hormonal cliff occurs at precisely the moment when a woman is expected to function at her highest capacity, with the least support, on the least sleep. The result, for vulnerable women, may be postpartum depression, postpartum anxiety, or in rare but devastating cases, postpartum psychosis. These conditions are not failures of maternal feeling; they are neurobiological events that require clinical intervention.

Perimenopause, the years preceding the final menstrual period, is a time of erratic hormonal fluctuation that is frequently misunderstood and frequently misdiagnosed. Estrogen levels do not decline steadily during perimenopause; they fluctuate unpredictably, sometimes reaching higher levels than during reproductive years before plummeting. This hormonal volatility produces symptoms that may be mistaken for primary psychiatric illness: mood instability, anxiety, irritability, insomnia, cognitive fog, and difficulty concentrating. The woman who has been psychiatrically stable for decades may suddenly find herself struggling, and she may attribute this to stress, aging, or personal failure rather than recognizing it as a biological transition. Clinicians who do not inquire about menstrual changes, vasomotor symptoms, and other markers of perimenopause will miss this diagnosis repeatedly.

Menopause itself—defined retrospectively as twelve months without menstruation—represents a new hormonal equilibrium. For some women, the end of hormonal fluctuation brings stability and relief. For others, the persistently low estrogen state produces ongoing symptoms that affect mood, cognition, and quality of life. The menopausal transition is not the end of a woman's psychiatric vulnerability; it is a reorganization that may require different approaches than those used in reproductive years.

Women do not simply "have disorders"—their symptoms interact with biology, identity, and circumstance in ways that require the clinician to think contextually. The question is not only what disorder is present, but when it emerged, how it relates to hormonal status, and how its presentation may shift across the phases of a woman's life.

II. The Weight Women Carry

Women's psychiatric presentations cannot be understood apart from the burdens they carry—burdens that are often invisible, often unacknowledged, and often assumed to be simply what women do. The cumulative weight of these burdens creates vulnerability to psychiatric illness and shapes how illness is experienced and expressed.

Emotional labor falls disproportionately on women. The work of tracking birthdays and managing social calendars, of sensing when a child is struggling or a partner is withdrawn, of maintaining relationships through attention and care, of anticipating needs and smoothing conflicts—this work is largely invisible and largely uncompensated, yet it is exhausting. The woman who appears to be doing nothing may be doing everything; the woman who is praised for holding the family together may be depleted by the effort of doing so.

Caregiving responsibilities extend in multiple directions. Women are more likely than men to be primary caregivers for children, and they are more likely to assume responsibility for aging parents as well. The "sandwich generation"—caring for children and elders simultaneously—is disproportionately female. These responsibilities are not merely time-consuming; they are emotionally demanding, often relentless, and frequently performed without adequate support. The woman who cannot understand why she is so exhausted may be carrying more than any one person can sustain.

Societal expectations of selflessness teach women that their own needs should come last. The good mother prioritizes her children. The good wife supports her husband. The good daughter cares for her parents. The good employee goes the extra mile. These expectations are often internalized so deeply that a woman may feel guilty for having needs at all, may apologize for taking up the clinician's time, may minimize her suffering because others have it worse. The woman who finally seeks help may arrive already convinced that she is making too much of too little.

Vulnerability to sexual trauma and coercion marks many women's lives. Sexual violence, harassment, and coercion are not rare events; they are common experiences that shape how women move through the world, how they relate to their bodies, and how they respond to authority figures, including clinicians. The woman in the consulting room may carry a trauma history she has never disclosed to anyone, may have symptoms she does not connect to what happened to her, may find the vulnerability of seeking help reactivating the helplessness of prior violation. The clinician who does not hold this possibility in mind will miss what is most important.

The pressure to remain functional regardless of internal distress creates a particular bind. Women are expected to keep going—to care for children, show up at work, maintain the household, support others—regardless of how they feel. This expectation is internalized: the depressed woman who can still function may tell herself she is not really sick; the anxious woman who manages to meet her obligations may not believe she deserves help. By the time a woman's symptoms are severe enough to overcome her own minimization and the minimization of those around her, she may be profoundly ill.

These burdens are not psychiatric diagnoses, but they create the conditions in which psychiatric illness flourishes. They shape presentation: the woman's depression may appear as exhaustion, her anxiety as irritability with her children, her trauma as inability to tolerate intimacy with her partner. And they shape treatment: the woman who is depleted by caregiving needs more than medication; she needs permission to have needs, space to meet them, and perhaps structural changes in her life that cannot be prescribed.

III. Diagnostic Complexity in Women

Psychiatric diagnosis in women is complicated by atypical presentations, by the overlay of hormonal factors, by the minimization of female distress, and by patterns of misdiagnosis that have affected generations of women.

Depression

Depression in women often presents differently than the textbook descriptions suggest. Sadness may be present, but it may be overshadowed by guilt—guilt about being a bad mother, a bad wife, a bad daughter, a bad employee, guilty for having needs, guilty for not being grateful, guilty for being depressed at all. Depletion may dominate the picture: the woman describes having nothing left, running on empty, dragging herself through days that feel endless. Irritability may be more prominent than sadness, manifesting as short temper with children, frustration with partners, inability to tolerate demands that previously felt manageable. Somatic symptoms—headaches, fatigue, pain, gastrointestinal distress—may be the primary complaint, leading to medical workups that reveal nothing while the underlying depression goes unrecognized. Cognitive fog—difficulty concentrating, forgetting words, losing track of tasks—may cause the woman to fear dementia when she is actually depressed.

The woman who presents saying she is "stressed" or "overwhelmed" may be depressed. The woman who presents for evaluation of chronic fatigue may be depressed. The woman who has been told by her physician that her symptoms are "just anxiety" may be depressed. Asking about mood is necessary but not sufficient; the clinician must listen for depression's many disguises.

Anxiety

Anxiety disorders are more common in women than in men, and they often have a particular character in women. Anxiety may be highly somatic, with physical symptoms—racing heart, shortness of breath, dizziness, gastrointestinal distress—dominating the picture. It may be ruminative, with endless mental rehearsal of past conversations, future catastrophes, possible mistakes, and imagined judgments. It may be chronic and pervasive, a background hum of worry that the woman has lived with so long she considers it normal.

Women with anxiety often function at high levels despite their suffering, which leads both themselves and others to underestimate how much they are struggling. The woman who appears competent and successful may be held together by enormous effort, sustained by anxiety that drives performance while eroding well-being. By the time she seeks help, she may be exhausted by decades of invisible struggle.

Trauma-Related Disorders

Trauma-related disorders are highly prevalent in women, reflecting both the frequency of traumatic exposure—particularly interpersonal and sexual trauma—and the particular vulnerabilities that trauma creates. Symptoms may emerge years or decades after the original trauma, often surfacing during life transitions: after childbirth, during perimenopause, following divorce, after the death of a parent who was also an abuser.

The woman may not recognize her symptoms as trauma related. She may have dissociated the memories so completely that she does not connect her current distress to her past. She may have been told that what happened was not that bad, that she should be over it by now, that her continued suffering is evidence of weakness or self-indulgence. She may minimize her own experience in ways that mirror how others minimize in the present and past.

Trauma in women frequently manifests as difficulty in relationships, problems with intimacy and trust, chronic hypervigilance that masquerades as anxiety, dissociative symptoms that are mistaken for inattention, and somatic symptoms that send her to specialist after specialist without relief. The clinician who does not ask about trauma—gently, non-intrusively, with patience for whatever the woman is ready to share—will miss an essential part of the story.

Attention-Deficit/Hyperactivity Disorder

ADHD in women is frequently underdiagnosed until adulthood or perimenopause, when compensatory strategies finally fail or hormonal changes unmask symptoms that were previously managed. Girls with ADHD are less likely than boys to be hyperactive and disruptive; they are more likely to be inattentive, disorganized, and dreamy in ways that are attributed to personality rather than recognized as disorder. The girl who struggles academically despite evident intelligence may be told she is not trying hard enough. The girl who is overwhelmed by organizational demands may develop anxiety and perfectionism as compensatory strategies. The woman who has managed through sheer effort for decades may finally decompensate when the demands of career, family, and perhaps peri-menopause exceed what effort alone can sustain.

The woman diagnosed with ADHD in her forties often experiences profound relief—finally, an explanation for decades of struggle, for the sense of being fundamentally different, for the shame of never quite managing what others seemed to manage effortlessly. The diagnosis reframes her history; treatment offers hope for her future.

Bipolar Disorder

Bipolar disorder in women is often misdiagnosed, typically as recurrent major depression or as personality disorder. The depressive episodes are what bring women to treatment; the hypomanic episodes may be experienced as recovery, as finally feeling like themselves, as periods of productivity and energy that are welcomed rather than questioned. The woman with undiagnosed bipolar II disorder may have received multiple trials of antidepressants, each producing initial improvement followed by relapse, mood instability, or emergence of mixed features. She may have been told she has treatment-resistant depression when, what she has is inadequately diagnosed bipolar disorder.

Careful questioning about lifetime history of elevated mood, decreased need for sleep, increased energy, and behavioral changes is essential. The question is not only whether the woman is currently depressed but whether she has ever experienced periods that might represent the other pole of a cycling illness.

The Importance of Context

Diagnosis in women requires the clinician to ask not only what symptoms are present but what has this woman been told about her symptoms—by doctors, by family members, by herself. Many women have been told that their suffering is normal ("all new mothers feel this way"), exaggerated ("you're too sensitive"), or characterological ("you've always been anxious"). They have been offered reassurance when they needed treatment, dismissal when they needed validation, and personality labels when they needed diagnosis.

The clinician must be prepared to see what others have missed, to name what has been minimized, and to offer treatment for conditions that have been overlooked or mischaracterized. This is diagnostic work, but it is also therapeutic: the experience of being accurately understood can itself be healing.

IV. Medication Considerations Across Hormonal Phases

Pharmacological treatment in women must be adapted to the hormonal context in which illness occurs. The same disorder may require different approaches depending on whether a woman is menstruating, pregnant, postpartum, perimenopausal, or post-menopausal. The clinician must understand these contexts and adjust treatment accordingly.

The Menstrual Cycle and Premenstrual Dysphoric Disorder

For women whose psychiatric symptoms are stable across the menstrual cycle, standard treatment approaches apply. For women, whose symptoms fluctuate with their cycle—worsening premenstrual phase and improving after menstruation—this pattern itself is diagnostically and therapeutically significant.

Premenstrual dysphoric disorder (PMDD) represents an abnormal sensitivity to normal hormonal fluctuations. The hormonal changes themselves are not pathological; the brain's response to them is. Symptoms include severe mood lability, irritability, depression, anxiety, and physical symptoms that emerge during the luteal phase and resolve within days of menstruation. The impairment can be profound, affecting relationships, work, and quality of life for one to two weeks of every month.

SSRIs are remarkably effective for PMDD, and they work rapidly —often within days rather than the weeks required for major depression. They can be used continuously, providing stable symptom control throughout the cycle, or intermittently, taken only during the luteal phase when symptoms would otherwise emerge. The choice between continuous and intermittent dosing depends on patient preference, symptom pattern, and tolerability. Some women prefer the simplicity of continuous dosing; others prefer to minimize medication exposure and find luteal-phase dosing sufficient.

Hormonal approaches represent an alternative or adjunctive strategy. Oral contraceptives that suppress ovulation can eliminate the hormonal fluctuations that trigger symptoms. Extended-cycle or continuous formulations that eliminate the hormone-free interval may be particularly effective. GnRH agonists can suppress ovarian function more completely, though their side effects and long-term implications limit their use to refractory cases.

For women with underlying psychiatric disorders that worsen premenstrually, addressing the premenstrual exacerbation may require dose adjustments during the luteal phase, the addition of an anxiolytic or sleep aid for the most symptomatic days, or optimization of the underlying treatment to provide greater stability across the cycle.

Pregnancy

Psychiatric illness during pregnancy presents a double bind: untreated illness carries real risks to mother and fetus, but medication exposure also carries potential risks. The clinician must help the woman navigate this uncertainty, providing information that allows her to make decisions aligned with her values while supporting whatever decision she makes.

Untreated depression during pregnancy is associated with poor prenatal care, inadequate nutrition, substance use, preterm delivery, low birth weight, and postpartum depression. Untreated anxiety is associated with increased stress hormones that may affect fetal development. Untreated bipolar disorder carries risks of mood episode during pregnancy or postpartum, with potentially devastating consequences. The alternative to medication is not a risk-free pregnancy; it is a pregnancy in which untreated illness poses its own dangers.

Medication risks vary by agent and by trimester. SSRIs as a class have reassuring reproductive safety data, though no medication can be declared absolutely safe. Sertraline has the most extensive data in pregnancy and is often preferred when starting or switching medications during pregnancy. Paroxetine has been associated with a small increased risk of cardiac malformations, leading many clinicians to avoid it in the first trimester or to switch women on paroxetine to alternative agents before conception when possible. SNRIs have less data than SSRIs but appear to have similar risk profiles.

Lithium carries a risk of cardiac malformations, particularly Ebstein's anomaly, though the absolute risk is lower than historically believed—about one to two per thousand rather than the much higher rates once reported. For women with severe bipolar disorder for whom lithium is essential, the decision may be to continue with careful fetal monitoring, including detailed cardiac ultrasonography. For women for whom alternatives exist, switching to agents with more reassuring data—lamotrigine, for example—may be preferred.

Valproate is contraindicated in pregnancy due to significant risks of neural tube defects and neurodevelopmental impairment. Women of reproductive potential taking valproate should be counseled about these risks and offered effective contraception or transition to alternative agents if pregnancy is possible.

Atypical antipsychotics have accumulating safety data that is generally reassuring, though long-term neurodevelopmental outcomes are still being studied. For women who require antipsychotic medication during pregnancy, continuing effective treatment is usually preferable to switching to unfamiliar agents or discontinuing treatment.

Benzodiazepines near delivery can produce neonatal sedation and, rarely, neonatal withdrawal syndrome. When benzodiazepines are necessary, using the lowest effective dose and tapering before delivery, when possible, can reduce these risks.

The decision about medication in pregnancy should be made collaboratively, with the woman as the primary decision-maker. The clinician's role is to provide accurate information about risks and benefits, to correct misconceptions, to support the woman's autonomy, and to ensure that whatever decision is made, she receives appropriate follow-up. Some women will choose to continue medication; some will choose to discontinue; some will choose to reduce doses or switch agents. Each of these decisions can be reasonable depending on the woman's circumstances, illness severity, prior history, and values.

The Postpartum Period

The postpartum period is a time of extreme psychiatric vulnerability. Postpartum depression affects ten to fifteen percent of women; postpartum anxiety is similarly common; postpartum psychosis, though rarer, is a psychiatric emergency that requires immediate intervention.

Postpartum depression often emerges insidiously during the first weeks or months after delivery. The woman may not recognize her symptoms as depression; she may attribute her exhaustion to the demands of newborn care, her irritability to sleep deprivation, her lack of enjoyment to the difficulty of the transition. She may feel guilty about not feeling the joy she expected, ashamed of her ambivalence toward her baby, terrified that her dark thoughts mean she is a bad mother. She may not disclose her symptoms because she fears judgment, fears having her baby taken away, fears confirming her own sense of failure.

Screening for postpartum depression should be routine, using validated instruments such as the Edinburgh Postnatal Depression Scale. Treatment should be initiated promptly when screening is positive and clinical evaluation confirms the diagnosis. SSRIs are effective and compatible with breastfeeding; sertraline is often preferred because of its minimal excretion into breast milk. The woman's preference about breastfeeding should be respected; if she prefers to breastfeed and a compatible medication is available, this should be supported; if she prefers to use formula in order to use a different medication or to have her partner share nighttime feeding, this too should be supported.

Brexanolone, a neurosteroid specifically approved for postpartum depression, represents a novel mechanism—modulation of GABA-A receptors—and produces rapid improvement, but it requires sixty hours of continuous intravenous infusion in a supervised setting, limiting its practical utility. Its existence as proof of concept has led to development of oral agents with similar mechanisms.

Postpartum anxiety may occur independently or alongside depression. The woman may experience intrusive thoughts about harm coming to her baby—what if she drops him, what if she forgets him, what if she hurts him. These thoughts are typically ego-dystonic, experienced as horrifying intrusions rather than desires, and they are associated with anxiety rather than intent. Reassurance that these thoughts are common and do not predict actual harm is essential; treatment with SSRIs addresses the underlying anxiety that generates them.

Postpartum psychosis is a psychiatric emergency. It typically emerges within the first two weeks after delivery and is characterized by confusion, disorganization, mood lability, delusions, and hallucinations. The risk of harm to self or infant is significant; hospitalization is usually necessary; treatment with antipsychotics, mood stabilizers, and sometimes electroconvulsive therapy produces rapid improvement in most cases. Women who have experienced postpartum psychosis have a high risk of recurrence with subsequent pregnancies and should be counseled about this risk and offered prophylactic treatment if they choose to become pregnant again.

Perimenopause

Perimenopause is a time of psychiatric vulnerability that is frequently misdiagnosed. The woman who has been psychiatrically stable for years may suddenly develop symptoms that seem to emerge from nowhere: anxiety that wakes her at night, mood swings that strain her relationships, cognitive fog that makes her fear early dementia, fatigue that no amount of sleep resolves.

These symptoms often have a hormonal basis. The erratic estrogen fluctuations of perimenopause affect serotonin, norepinephrine, and other neurotransmitter systems. Vasomotor symptoms—hot flashes and night sweats—disrupt sleep, and sleep disruption destabilizes mood. The woman may attribute her symptoms to stress, to aging, to personal weakness, not recognizing that her brain is responding to a biological transition.

Treatment must address both the psychiatric symptoms and their hormonal context. SSRIs and SNRIs are effective for perimenopausal mood and anxiety symptoms, and some—particularly venlafaxine, desvenlafaxine, and paroxetine—also reduce vasomotor symptoms. For women whose symptoms are clearly linked to hormonal fluctuation, hormone therapy may be beneficial, though decisions about hormone therapy must weigh psychiatric benefits against other medical considerations. Gabapentin can address both anxiety and vasomotor symptoms. Clonidine provides another non-hormonal option for hot flashes.

The perimenopausal woman deserves validation that her symptoms are real, that they have a biological basis, and that they are treatable. She is not imagining things; she is not "just stressed"; she is not weak. She is experiencing a biological transition that affects her brain, and she deserves treatment that addresses what is actually happening.

Menopause

Menopause, once established, represents a new hormonal steady state. For some women, the end of hormonal fluctuation brings stability and relief. For others, the persistently low estrogen state continues to affect mood, cognition, and quality of life.

Treatment approaches in postmenopausal women are generally similar to those in other populations, with attention to considerations that become more relevant with age: cognitive effects of medications, drug interactions with treatments for other medical conditions, metabolic and cardiovascular risks, and bone health. Some medications that are well-tolerated in younger women become problematic in older women; anticholinergic effects, for example, may produce cognitive impairment that was not apparent at younger ages.

The postmenopausal woman may have decades of life ahead of her. Treatment that is effective and tolerable supports her continued engagement with work, relationships, creativity, and meaning.

V. Trauma, Autonomy, and the Therapeutic Alliance

Many women have learned, through long experience, to minimize their own needs. They have been taught that their feelings are too much, that their suffering is less important than others', that their role is to care for them rather than to receive care. This learning shapes how they present for treatment and what they need from the clinician.

A therapeutic alliance that restores autonomy and validates suffering is essential. The woman who has been dismissed, minimized, and disbelieved needs a clinician who listens, who takes her seriously, who treats her symptoms as worthy of attention and her suffering as worthy of relief. This is not mere kindness; it is therapeutic. The experience of being believed and respected may itself initiate healing.

Shared decision-making is not optional in treating women—it is therapeutic. The woman who has felt controlled, who has had choices made for her, who has learned that her preferences do not matter, needs a treatment relationship in which her voice is central. The clinician who presents options rather than dictates, who explains reasoning rather than pronounces conclusions, who asks what the woman prefers and responds to her answer, provides more than good care; the clinician provides a corrective experience that may help heal wounds older than the current illness.

Trauma-informed care is essential for many women, whether or not their presenting symptoms are explicitly trauma-related. The woman who has experienced sexual trauma may find the vulnerability of the clinical encounter reactivating; she may need more control over the physical space, the pace of disclosure, and the structure of treatment. The woman who has experienced violations of autonomy may be exquisitely sensitive to any hint of coercion. The woman who has been gaslighted may need repeated validation that what she perceives is real.

The clinician must be prepared to meet each woman where she is, to provide safety without demanding disclosure, to support autonomy without abandoning clinical guidance, and to offer treatment that respects both her vulnerability and her strength.

. . .

VI. Substance Use in Women

Substance use in women often occurs privately, hidden from partners, families, and clinicians. The woman who drinks alone after the children are in bed, the woman who uses cannabis to quiet her racing mind, the woman who relies on stimulants obtained from a friend to manage demands that exceed her capacity—these patterns may go undetected for years.

Women often use substances as self-medication for symptoms that have not been otherwise addressed. Alcohol provides anxiolysis and sleep induction; cannabis offers relief from anxiety and from intrusive thoughts; stimulants enable function despite exhaustion and attentional difficulties. What begins as occasional use may progress to dependence, and the progression can be rapid. Women develop alcohol-related liver disease faster than men; they progress from first use to dependence more quickly; they face greater stigma when their substance use becomes known.

Shame delays disclosure. The woman who drinks too much knows she is not supposed to; the mother who uses substances feels she is failing her children; the professional woman fears what acknowledgment would mean for her career and reputation. She may minimize her use even to her clinician, offering partial truths that obscure the extent of the problem.

Compassionate inquiry is essential. The clinician must ask about substance use directly, routinely, without judgment. The woman must feel that disclosure will be met with understanding rather than condemnation, with treatment rather than punishment. When substance use is present, it must be integrated into the treatment plan —not as a moral failing but as a clinical issue requiring clinical intervention.

.   .   .

VII. Clinical Illustrations

Perimenopausal Unraveling

A forty-seven-year-old woman presented convinced that she was developing early-onset dementia. For several months, she had experienced difficulty concentrating, word-finding problems, forgotten appointments, and a mental fog that made her previously sharp mind feel dull. She was irritable with her husband and teenage children in ways that distressed her. She was sleeping poorly, waking multiple times a night feeling overheated. She was anxious in ways she had never been, her mind churning with worries she could not quiet.

Her periods had become irregular over the past year—sometimes early, sometimes late, sometimes heavy, sometimes barely present. She had not connected this to her cognitive and emotional symptoms; she had assumed the menstrual changes were simply aging while the psychiatric symptoms were something more ominous.

The diagnosis was perimenopause, not dementia. Her symptoms — the cognitive fog, mood lability, sleep disruption, and the anxiety —were all consistent with the erratic estrogen fluctuations of the menopausal transition. Neuropsychological testing was normal, confirming what the clinical picture suggested.

An SNRI addressed both her mood symptoms and her vasomotor symptoms; the night sweats improved within weeks, and as her sleep improved, her cognition cleared. She was not losing her mind; she was going through a transition that had neuropsychiatric manifestations. Understanding this reframed her experience: she was not failing, she was not deteriorating, she was changing in ways that were biological, predictable, and treatable.

Postpartum Descent

A new mother in her early thirties presented six weeks after delivery with severe anxiety that had been dismissed by her obstetrician as "normal new-mother worries." She was not sleeping even when the baby slept; she lay awake monitoring his breathing, checking, and rechecking that he was still alive. She had intrusive thoughts about terrible things happening to him—what if she fell down the stairs while carrying him, what if she left him in the car, what if she smothered him accidentally while nursing.

These thoughts horrified her. She was certain they meant she was a danger to her baby, that some part of her wanted to harm him, that she was a monster. She had told no one about the thoughts because she feared her baby would be taken away.

What she was experiencing was postpartum anxiety with intrusive thoughts—not uncommon, not predictive of actual harm, and highly treatable. The thoughts were symptoms, not intentions; they emerged from anxiety, not desire; they indicated that she cared desperately about her baby, not that she was a danger to him.

An SSRI reduced anxiety and with it the intrusive thoughts. Psychoeducation about the nature of intrusive thoughts relieved her terror that she was capable of harming her child. Within weeks, she was sleeping when the baby slept, enjoying moments of connection with him, feeling like herself again.

Early treatment protected both mother and infant—not only from the immediate suffering but from the longer-term consequences of untreated postpartum illness: impaired bonding, developmental effects on the child, risk of chronic or recurrent depression, and damage to the marriage that was already strained by the new demands of parenthood.

Sexual Trauma, Long Silent

A professional woman in her fifties presented for treatment of depression that had not responded adequately to multiple medication trials. She was accomplished, articulate, and apparently put-together; she described her symptoms clearly and provided a thorough history—but something felt incomplete.

After several months of treatment, during which her depression improved somewhat but her sleep remained disturbed and she remained hypervigilant in ways that seemed disproportionate to her current life, she disclosed that she had been sexually abused by a family member throughout her childhood. She had never told anyone. She had walled off those years so completely that she rarely thought about them consciously, but she recognized that she had never felt safe, never trusted easily, never fully inhabited her body.

The disclosure changed the treatment. Her symptoms made new sense as a trauma sequela rather than treatment-resistant depression. Her medication was not stopped, but the focus of treatment expanded to include trauma-informed therapy, at her own pace, with her in control of what she disclosed and when.

What mattered most, she said later, was not any particular intervention. What mattered was that she was validated. She had spent her life convinced that if she told, she would not be believed—or that she would be blamed, that it would be her fault, that she had somehow caused what had been done to her. The experience of telling her story and being met with belief, with compassion, with recognition of the profound violation she had survived-this was therapeutic in ways that no medication could replicate.

ADHD Recognized Late

A capable woman in her mid-forties presented for evaluation at the suggestion of her daughter, who had recently been diagnosed with ADHD and who saw her own symptoms reflected in her mother's lifelong struggles. The woman had always been "scattered"—losing things, running late, starting projects she didn't finish, feeling overwhelmed by organizational demands that others seemed to manage effortlessly. She had compensated through sheer effort, through the anxiety that drove her to check and recheck, through elaborate systems that partially contained her disorganization.

The diagnosis of ADHD reframed her life. The struggles she had attributed to personal failing-to not trying hard enough, not caring enough, not being as smart as she seemed—were symptoms of a neurobiological condition. She was not lazy; she was not stupid; she was not morally defective. She had a disorder, and it was treatable.

Stimulant medication produced immediate improvement in focus, organization, and follow-through. Tasks that had previously required enormous effort became manageable. The mental noise quieted. She could think in straight lines rather than circles.

But the medication was only part of what mattered. The larger transformation was in her self-understanding. Decades of shame dissolved as she recognized that she had been struggling against a brain that worked differently, not failing through lack of will. Self-compassion replaced self-condemnation. She grieved for the years of unnecessary suffering, then turned toward a future in which she could finally function as she had always wanted to.

VIII. Medication Approaches in Women

Pharmacological treatment in women follows the same principles as in other populations, but the application of these principles must be tailored to the biological and contextual factors that shape women's experience of illness and treatment.

Hormonal Context as Diagnostic Information

Incorporating hormonal stage into diagnosis is essential. The woman presenting with new psychiatric symptoms should be asked about her menstrual cycle, her pregnancy history, her menopausal status, and the relationship between hormonal changes and symptom onset or exacerbation. This information shapes diagnosis, prognosis, and treatment selection. The depression that emerged during perimenopause may require different treatment than the depression that has been present since adolescence; the anxiety that worsens premenstrually may benefit from interventions targeted to that phase.

Trauma Screening

Screening for trauma history should be part of every comprehensive evaluation. The screening need not be intrusive; a simple question—"Many people have experiences in their past that still affect them. Is there anything from your past that you think is relevant to what you're experiencing now?"—opens the door without forcing entry. If the woman is not ready to disclose, the question establishes that the clinician is willing to hear; if she is ready, it provides the invitation she has been waiting for.

Perimenopause as a Neurobiological Transition

Treating perimenopause as a neurobiological transition rather than dismissing it as "just hormones" validates women's experience and opens the door to effective treatment. The perimenopausal woman whose symptoms are attributed to stress and aging receives neither validation nor relief; the woman whose symptoms are recognized as having a biological basis can receive treatment that addresses their origin.

Bipolarity Screening

Monitoring for bipolarity when prescribing antidepressants is particularly important in women, given the frequency with which bipolar disorder is misdiagnosed as recurrent depression. Before starting an antidepressant, the clinician should inquire about lifetime history of elevated mood, decreased need for sleep, increased energy, and other features of hypomania or mania. If bipolarity is present, antidepressant monotherapy carries risks of mood destabilization, rapid cycling, or mixed episodes; treatment should involve mood stabilization as the foundation.

Postpartum Illness as Urgent

Treating postpartum illness urgently protects both mother and child. Delays in treatment extend suffering, impair bonding, and risk progression to more severe illness. The woman with postpartum depression deserves rapid access to effective treatment, not a waiting list; the woman with postpartum psychosis requires immediate intervention, not observation.

Substance Use Assessment

Addressing substance use gently and directly acknowledges the reality that many women use substances to manage symptoms, that shame creates barriers to disclosure, and that compassionate inquiry is more effective than judgmental questioning. When substance use is present, it must be integrated into treatment rather than addressed as a separate issue or treated as a reason to withhold psychiatric care.

Shared Decision-Making

Using shared decision-making to restore autonomy is not merely good clinical practice; it is therapeutic, particularly for women whose autonomy has been violated or overridden. The woman who participates actively in treatment decisions, whose preferences are respected, whose questions are answered, and whose choices are supported experiences treatment as empowering rather than controlling.

Medication Selection

When selecting medications for women, the clinician should consider the specific factors that affect tolerability and safety in this population. Sexual side effects, though often discussed in the context of men, also affect women and can impair relationships and quality of life. Weight gain may be particularly distressing for women and may lead to non-adherence. Bone health becomes increasingly relevant as women age, and some medications may increase fracture risk.

For depression in women, SSRIs and SNRIs remain first-line treatments. Mirtazapine may be useful when insomnia and appetite suppression are prominent, though weight gain limits its use in some women. Bupropion offers an alternative when sexual side effects or weight gain must be avoided. For women with perimenopausal symptoms, SNRIs may provide dual benefit for mood and vasomotor symptoms.

For anxiety, SSRIs are effective and well-tolerated. Buspirone provides an alternative without sedation or dependence risk. Gabapentin may address both anxiety and vasomotor symptoms in perimenopausal women.

For ADHD in women, stimulant medications are effective and generally well-tolerated. The woman diagnosed in midlife may respond dramatically to treatment, finally experiencing what organized, focused attention feels like. Atomoxetine provides a non-stimulant alternative.

For bipolar disorder, lamotrigine is often preferred in women because of its effectiveness for bipolar depression, its tolerability, and its relatively favorable reproductive safety profile compared to valproate. Lithium remains an important option, particularly for women with suicidal ideation, though its use in pregnancy requires careful consideration. Valproate should generally be avoided in women of reproductive potential given the risks of fetal harm.

For insomnia, melatonin and cognitive-behavioral therapy for insomnia (CBT-I) are preferred over benzodiazepines and traditional hypnotics. Trazodone at low doses may be useful as an adjunct. For women with trauma-related nightmares, prazosin can reduce nightmare frequency and improve sleep quality.

. . .

IX. Closing Reflection

To treat women wisely is to see the whole terrain—the biology, the burdens, the resilience, and the stories carried quietly for years. Psychopharmacology becomes not merely intervention, but recognition and restoration.

Women's lives are marked by transitions that men do not experience—the monthly rhythm of the menstrual cycle, the transformation of pregnancy and childbirth, the reorganization of perimenopause and menopause. These transitions are not merely hormonal; they are existential, reshaping identity, relationships, and relationship to one's own body. Psychiatric illness interweaves with these transitions, emerging or remitting, worsening, or improving, taking forms shaped by the hormonal context in which it occurs.

Women's lives are marked by burdens that are often invisible— the emotional labor that maintains families, the caregiving that extends in every direction, the pressure to appear competent and self-less regardless of internal distress. These burdens are not psychiatric diagnoses, but they create the conditions in which illness flourishes and shape how illness is experienced and expressed.

Women's lives are marked by strengths that are often unseen— the resilience that survives trauma, the capacity to maintain function despite suffering, the ability to care for others while receiving little care. These strengths are resources for treatment, and they deserve acknowledgment even as the suffering that accompanies them is addressed.

The clinician who treats women must learn to see all of this: the biology and the biography, the symptoms and the context, the illness, and the identity. Medication is one tool among many, but it is a tool that can provide relief when relief has been long denied, stability when stability has been out of reach, and the capacity to engage with life when illness has made engagement impossible.

To treat women wisely is to offer this relief without diminishing the complexity of women's lives, to provide intervention without reducing women to their disorders, and to support healing that extends beyond symptom remission to restoration of agency, autonomy, and wholeness.

∼

PART IV

Some patients do not fit neatly into protocols. Their conditions cross boundaries — immunological, neurological, social, existential. Part IV addresses the edges of psychiatric practice: special populations, emerging science, the enduring role of psychotherapy, and the art of prescribing with wisdom rather than reflex.

11

SPECIAL POPULATIONS
WHERE DIAGNOSIS MEETS HUMANITY

P sychopharmacology reaches its greatest ethical and clinical complexity when it enters the lives of those who exist at the margins—socially, medically, culturally, or psychologically. These are the patients whose suffering is amplified by context, whose symptoms are filtered through trauma, disadvantage, or difference, and whose treatment requires not only knowledge but humility. To prescribe for these patients is to confront the limits of textbook medicine and to recognize that healing cannot be separated from history, environment, power, and meaning.

"Special populations" are not special because they are rare. They are special because standard approaches often fail them. The treatment algorithms developed in clinical trials enrolling stable, housed, insured patients with single diagnoses may not translate to the veteran whose hypervigilance is a survival adaptation, the autistic adult whose sensory sensitivities make standard medication doses intolerable, the refugee whose depression speaks through somatic idioms unfamiliar to Western medicine, or the formerly incarcerated patient whose treatment history has been repeatedly disrupted by forces beyond their control.

In these populations, medication decisions cannot be separated from the contexts in which patients live. What seem like pathological symptoms may actually be adaptive responses to extreme conditions. Nonadherence that appears irrational may represent wisdom born of experience—with medications that caused harm, with providers who did not listen, with systems that punished vulnerability. Resistance that appears oppositional may reflect a lifetime of having choices made by others, of being controlled rather than cared for, of surviving by refusing to surrender agency.

The clinician who treats special populations must bring not only pharmacological expertise but also cultural humility, trauma awareness, and willingness to question assumptions. The question is never simply what medication to prescribe but how to offer treatment in ways that respect autonomy, acknowledge history, and support healing in contexts where healing has often been denied.

I. TRAUMA SURVIVORS: When the Nervous System Never Learned Safety

Trauma reshapes the brain. The nervous system that has experienced overwhelming threat does not simply return to baseline when the threat passes; it reorganizes around the expectation of danger, maintaining vigilance long after vigilance is no longer necessary. This reorganization affects arousal systems, attention, sleep architecture, emotional regulation, interpersonal trust, and the very sense of inhabiting one's own body. Trauma is not merely a psychological experience; it is a neurobiological alteration that persists in circuits and symptoms.

The trauma survivor may present with hypervigilance that appears as anxiety, with emotional numbing that appears as depression, with irritability that appears as anger dysregulation, with dissociation that appears as inattention, with substance use that appears as addiction, with somatic symptoms that appear as medical illness. The presenting complaint may bear little obvious relationship to the underlying trauma; the patient may not connect their current suffering to what happened years or decades ago; the trauma itself may be fragmented, dissociated, or never disclosed. The clinician who takes symptoms at face value, who treats the anxiety without inquiring about its origins, who prescribes to help insomnia without understanding what the patient fears when they close their eyes, will provide incomplete care at best and retraumatizing care at worst.

UNDERSTANDING TRAUMA'S **Neurobiological Legacy**

Chronic exposure to threat alters the stress response systems in ways that persist long after the threat has ended. The hypothalamic-pituitary-adrenal axis, which regulates cortisol release in response to stress, may become dysregulated—either hyperresponsive, flooding the system with stress hormones at minor provocations, or hyporesponsive, reflecting exhaustion of the stress response after years of chronic activation. The amygdala, which detects threat, may become hypersensitive, triggering alarm responses to stimuli that objectively pose no danger. The prefrontal cortex, which normally modulates amygdala activity and supports rational appraisal of threat, may function less effectively, leaving the survivor at the mercy of automatic fear responses they cannot override through reason.

Sleep is particularly affected. The trauma survivor may be unable to sleep because sleep requires letting down one's guard, because nightmares make sleep itself threatening, because the transition to sleep feels like a loss of control that echoes the helplessness of the original trauma. The hyper-aroused nervous system that served survival during the trauma now prevents the rest that is essential for recovery. Sleep deprivation, in turn, worsens emotional regulation, cognitive function, and capacity to benefit from psychotherapy.

Dissociation—the disconnection from one's own experience, body, or sense of continuous identity—represents another adaptation to overwhelming threat. When escape is impossible and resistance is futile, the mind can escape by separating from the experience, by going somewhere else while the body endures what cannot be stopped. This capacity for dissociation, once developed, may persist, and activate in response to reminders of trauma, to stress, or even to the intensity of therapeutic work. The dissociative patient may appear present but not really present; may hear what is said but not register it; may agree to treatment plans they cannot later recall.

Clinical Principles in Treating Trauma Survivors

Prioritizing safety and predictability are the foundation of trauma-informed care. The trauma survivor's nervous system is organized around the expectation of danger; healing requires experiences that gradually teach safety. In the clinical encounter, this means consistency—keeping appointments, starting on time, avoiding surprises. It means transparency—explaining what you are doing and why, warning before physical examination, checking in about comfort. It means attention to the physical environment—ensuring the patient can see the door, asking about seating preferences, being aware that small spaces or certain smells may be triggering.

Treating sleep early is essential. Sleep deprivation worsens every psychiatric symptom and impairs the emotional processing that is essential for trauma recovery. Yet sleep is often among the most difficult symptoms to address in trauma survivors because the approaches that work for ordinary insomnia—relaxation, letting go of vigilance, surrendering to unconsciousness—are precisely what the traumatized nervous system resists. Prazosin, an alpha-1 adrenergic antagonist, can reduce nightmares and improve sleep quality in PTSD by dampening the noradrenergic arousal that drives trauma-related dreams. Trazodone may provide sedation without the dependence risk of benzodiazepines. Mirtazapine addresses both insomnia and depression. The goal is to make sleep safe enough that the patient can begin to get the rest their nervous system needs.

SSRIs and SNRIs remain first-line pharmacological treatments for PTSD and trauma-related disorders. Sertraline and paroxetine are FDA-approved for PTSD; other SSRIs and the SNRIs venlafaxine and duloxetine also have evidence of efficacy. These medications reduce hyperarousal, improve emotional regulation, and may facilitate engagement with trauma-focused psychotherapy. They do not erase trauma or eliminate all symptoms, but they can lower the baseline level of distress enough that the patient can begin to do the psychological work of processing what happened.

Mood stabilizers may be useful when emotional dysregulation is prominent—when the patient experiences intense, rapidly shifting emotions, when irritability or anger are difficult to control, when impulsiveness leads to self-destructive behavior. The mood lability of complex trauma can resemble bipolar disorder; the distinction matters for treatment selection, though the boundaries are often unclear. Lamotrigine, valproate, and some atypical antipsychotics may help stabilize affect, though evidence specifically in trauma populations is limited.

Avoiding medications that replicate helplessness is a critical principle that is often overlooked. Benzodiazepines may seem appealing for the hyper-aroused, anxious trauma survivor—they provide rapid relief and can feel like rescue. But benzodiazepines impair memory consolidation in ways that may interfere with trauma processing; they create dependence that can replicate the dynamics of abusive relationships; they produce discontinuation symptoms that may be experienced as loss of control; and they can worsen dissociation and emotional numbing. For most trauma survivors, benzodiazepines should be avoided or used only briefly and cautiously. Similarly, medications that produce sedation, cognitive dulling, or a sense of being controlled may be particularly distressing to patients whose traumatic experiences involved loss of agency.

Integrating psychotherapy is essential. Medication alone is insufficient treatment for trauma-related disorders. Trauma-focused cognitive-behavioral therapy, eye movement desensitization and reprocessing (EMDR), cognitive processing therapy, and prolonged exposure all have strong evidence for efficacy. These treatments help patients process traumatic memories, develop new narratives about what happened, and learn that reminders of trauma can be tolerated without catastrophe. Medication should support this work—by reducing symptoms enough that the patient can engage, by stabilizing mood and sleep, by modulating arousal—but medication cannot replace it.

The Meaning of Symptoms

In trauma survivors, symptoms often carry meaning beyond their phenomenology. The hypervigilance that appears as anxiety was once necessary for survival; the emotional numbing that appears as depression was once the only way to endure unbearable feelings; the dissociation that appears as detachment was once an escape when no other escape was possible. These adaptations, however costly in the present, were once solutions. Treating them as mere pathology, as errors to be corrected, misses their significance.

The clinician who can see symptoms as once as adaptive

responses communicates something important to the patient: that their survival strategies were intelligent, that they did what they needed to do, that their suffering is not evidence of weakness but of having survived what should not have been survived. This perspective does not preclude treatment—the goal is still to reduce suffering and improve function—but it changes the therapeutic relationship. The patient is not broken and in need of repair; they are carrying adaptations that were once necessary and are now ready to be released.

II. Neurodevelopmental Disorders: Across the Lifespan

Attention-deficit/hyperactivity disorder and autism spectrum disorder are typically discussed as conditions of childhood, but they are lifelong conditions whose manifestations change across development. Many adults with these conditions were never diagnosed in childhood—because they were girls, because they compensated effectively, because their presentation did not match stereotyped expectations, because the diagnostic concepts themselves were less developed in earlier decades. These adults arrive in adulthood carrying years of struggle, often with secondary psychiatric conditions, often with internalized narratives of failure and deficiency, often with profound relief when they finally receive an accurate diagnosis.

ADHD in Adults

Adult ADHD is frequently both underdiagnosed and, in certain settings, over diagnosed. Underdiagnosis often occurs in individuals who have compensated for their symptoms through intelligence, diligence, or anxiety, while overdiagnosis may result when symptoms of other conditions are incorrectly attributed to attentional difficulties. The core features of ADHD persist in adulthood but often manifest differently than in childhood. Hyperactivity may become internal restlessness rather than running and climbing; inattention may manifest as difficulty sustaining focus in meetings rather than failure to complete homework; impulsivity may appear as interrupting conversations or making impetuous decisions rather than blurting out answers in class.

The adult with undiagnosed ADHD has typically developed an array of compensatory strategies—calendars and reminders, anxiety-driven checking, and rechecking, choosing careers that match their strengths, relying on partners who provide external structure. These strategies may work well enough that the diagnosis is not obvious, but they come at a cost. The effort required to function may be exhausting; the anxiety that drives compensation may itself become impairing; the accumulation of failures—lost jobs, failed relationships, unfulfilled potential—may produce depression and demoralization that overshadow the underlying ADHD.

Stimulant medications remain the most effective treatment for ADHD across the lifespan. In adults, as in children, methylphenidate and amphetamine derivatives improve attention, reduce impulsivity, and enhance executive function. The response rate is high, and when the diagnosis is correct, the improvement can be transformative. An adult who has struggled for decades to focus, to complete tasks, to follow through on intentions may find that stimulant medication allows them to function in ways they never could before.

The emotional benefits of treatment are often as significant as the cognitive benefits. ADHD is not merely a disorder of attention; it involves emotional dysregulation, rejection sensitivity, and difficulty modulating affective responses. Stimulant medication often improves emotional regulation along with cognitive function, reducing the hair-trigger reactivity and emotional intensity that complicate relationships and self-image.

Treatment of adult ADHD reduces the risk of substance use disorders. Untreated ADHD is a significant risk factor for substance use, and stimulant treatment appears to be protective rather than a gateway to addiction. The adult with untreated ADHD may have been self-medicating with caffeine, nicotine, cannabis, or other substances for years; effective treatment of the underlying condition often reduces the drive toward self-medication.

Non-stimulant options exist for adults who cannot tolerate stimulants or for whom stimulants are contraindicated. Atomoxetine, a norepinephrine reuptake inhibitor, improves ADHD symptoms though less dramatically than stimulants. Bupropion has modest efficacy and may be useful when depression and ADHD coexist. Viloxazine, approved more recently, provides another non-stimulant option. Alpha-2 agonists such as guanfacine may help with emotional dysregulation and impulsivity though they are less effective for core attentional symptoms.

Autism in Adults

Autism spectrum disorder in adults is frequently unrecognized, particularly in those who have learned to mask their autistic traits through conscious effort and social imitation. Women and girls have historically been underdiagnosed because their presentations often differ from the stereotyped male presentation—they may have stronger social motivation, more effective masking, and special interests that are more socially typical. Adults who were not diagnosed in childhood may have received a variety of other diagnoses—anxiety, depression, social phobia, personality disorders—that captured pieces of their experience without explaining the whole.

The core features of autism—differences in social communication, restricted and repetitive patterns of behavior and interest, sensory sensitivities—persist across the lifespan, though their manifestation changes with development and the demands of adult life.

The autistic adult may have learned the rules of social interaction intellectually but find social engagement exhausting because it requires constant conscious effort. They may have intense interests that provide deep satisfaction but that others find unusual or excessive. They may experience sensory environments that others find unremarkable—fluorescent lights, background noise, certain textures —as overwhelming or painful.

Medication for autism addresses co-occurring conditions rather than autism itself. There is no medication that treats the core features of autism, nor is it clear that treating those features as pathology is the right framework. But many autistic adults have co-occurring anxiety, depression, ADHD, or other conditions that are appropriate targets for pharmacological treatment.

Autistic individuals may be highly sensitive to medications, experiencing side effects at lower doses than typically expected. Starting low and titrating slowly is particularly important in this population. Sensory sensitivities may extend to the physical experience of taking medication-the texture of tablets, the taste of liquids, the sensation of capsules swallowing. These concerns should be taken seriously and accommodated when possible.

The correct diagnosis often relieves shame more than medication alone. The autistic adult who has spent decades feeling fundamentally different, wrong, or broken may experience profound relief in learning that they have a recognizable neurological difference—that their struggles have a name, that others share their experience, that they are not alone. This reframing of identity, from failure to neurodivergence, can be more therapeutic than any medication. The clinician's role is not merely to diagnose but to provide this reframing in a way that the patient can receive—validating their experience, connecting them with resources and community, and supporting the process of integrating this new understanding into their sense of self.

. . .

III. Chronic Medical Illness: Mind and Body Entwined

Patients with chronic medical illness face challenges that are simultaneously physical and psychological, and the distinction between the two is often artificial. The pain of rheumatoid arthritis, the fatigue of heart failure, the uncertainty of cancer, the limitations of multiple sclerosis—these are not merely physical symptoms to which patients have psychological reactions. They are experiences that reshape identity, alter relationships, challenge meaning, and transform the felt sense of inhabiting a body.

Depression and anxiety are not simply common in chronic medical illness; they are intrinsic to the experience of living with a body that does not work as it should. The rates of depression in chronic illness far exceed those in the general population—reaching thirty to forty percent in conditions such as heart failure, stroke, and cancer. Yet these psychiatric conditions are frequently underdiagnosed and undertreated, dismissed as understandable reactions to difficult circumstances rather than recognized as treatable conditions that worsen medical outcomes and reduce quality of life.

The Bidirectional Relationship

The relationship between chronic medical illness and psychiatric symptoms is bidirectional. Medical illness causes psychiatric symptoms through multiple mechanisms: direct effects on the brain, inflammatory processes that affect mood, pain that disrupts sleep and function, medication side effects, and the psychological impact of loss and limitation. Psychiatric symptoms worsen medical illness through equally multiple mechanisms: nonadherence to treatment, unhealthy behaviors, physiological effects of chronic stress, and impaired engagement with medical care.

This bidirectional relationship means that treating psychiatric symptoms is not merely supportive care; it is disease-modifying. Treating depression in patients who have had myocardial infarction improves cardiac outcomes. Treating depression in diabetes improves glycemic control. Treating anxiety and depression in cancer patients improves quality of life and may improve survival. Psychiatric treatment is not separate from the medical treatment; it is part of it.

The Challenge of Invalidation

Patients with chronic illness often face a particular form of suffering that comes from not being believed—by doctors who minimize their symptoms, by family members who grow tired of their limitations, by disability systems that question their claims, by a culture that values productivity and views chronic illness as failure. This invalidation compounds the suffering of the illness itself, adding shame and isolation to pain and limitation.

The woman with fibromyalgia whose doctors have implied that her pain is not real, the man with chronic fatigue syndrome whose family wonders if he is simply lazy, the patient with multiple chemical sensitivity who is treated as a hypochondriac—these patients arrive at psychiatric evaluation already defended, already anticipating dismissal, already uncertain whether they will be believed. The clinician's first task is to validate their suffering, to communicate clearly that their symptoms are real, that their distress is warranted, and that they deserve treatment. This validation is itself therapeutic; it creates the possibility of a trusting relationship in which treatment can proceed.

Pharmacological Considerations in Chronic Medical Illness

Medication selection in chronic medical illness requires attention to factors that may not apply in otherwise healthy patients. Organ function affects drug metabolism and elimination; renal impairment may require dose reduction or avoidance of renally cleared medications; hepatic impairment affects the metabolism of many psychotropics. Polypharmacy increases the risk of drug-drug interactions, and patients with chronic illness are often taking multiple medications with which psychiatric drugs may interact.

Certain medications serve dual purposes in medically ill patients, addressing both psychiatric and medical symptoms. SNRIs such as duloxetine can treat depression while also providing analgesia for neuropathic pain and fibromyalgia. Mirtazapine can treat depression while also stimulating appetite and reducing nausea, useful in patients with cancer or wasting conditions. Gabapentin and pregabalin can address both anxiety and neuropathic pain. These dual-purpose medications allow more efficient treatment with fewer total medications, reducing pill burden and interaction risk.

Inflammation, increasingly recognized as a factor in depression, is common in chronic medical illness. Conditions characterized by chronic inflammation—autoimmune diseases, heart failure, chronic infections—may produce depression through inflammatory mechanisms that are partially distinct from the neurotransmitter abnormalities targeted by conventional antidepressants. Whether anti-inflammatory approaches have a role in treating depression in medically ill patients remains an area of investigation.

Sleep disruption is nearly universal in chronic medical illness—caused by pain, by medication effects, by sleep apnea, by nocturia, by the disruption of normal routines that illness imposes. Addressing sleep is essential, both because sleep deprivation worsens psychiatric symptoms and because adequate sleep is necessary for medical recovery and coping. The approach to insomnia in medically ill patients must consider the underlying causes—treating pain, adjusting medication timing, evaluating for sleep apnea—rather than simply adding hypnotics.

Fatigue is similarly complex in chronic medical illness. It may reflect depression, but it may also reflect the medical illness itself, medication side effects, sleep disruption, or deconditioning. Distinguishing depressive fatigue from illness-related fatigue is often impossible; the two are intertwined. Treatment of depression may improve fatigue; treatment of the underlying medical condition may improve both. Stimulants are sometimes used for fatigue in medically ill patients, particularly in cancer and palliative care settings, though evidence for their efficacy is limited.

IV. Incarcerated and Formerly Incarcerated Individuals

The intersection of mental illness and incarceration represents one of the great failures of contemporary American society. Jails and prisons have become de facto psychiatric institutions, housing more people with serious mental illness than all psychiatric hospitals combined. The prevalence of psychiatric conditions in incarcerated populations far exceeds that in the general population: depression, bipolar disorder, PTSD, schizophrenia, and substance use disorders are all vastly overrepresented. Many incarcerated individuals have untreated ADHD that contributed to the impulsive behaviors that led to their incarceration. Trauma histories are nearly universal.

The conditions of incarceration often exacerbate psychiatric illness. Isolation, violence, lack of privacy, unpredictability, and powerlessness worsen symptoms of PTSD and depression. Solitary confinement produces profound psychological deterioration, including psychosis, even in previously healthy individuals. Access to psychiatric care is often limited, continuity is poor, and medications may be abruptly discontinued or changed when patients are transferred between facilities.

The Challenges of Continuity

The incarcerated patient faces constant disruption of care. Transfer between facilities, release from incarceration, and gaps in insurance coverage all create discontinuities that interrupt treatment and increase relapse risk. The patient who was stable on medication while incarcerated may lose access to that medication on release; the patient who established a therapeutic relationship with a provider may be transferred to a facility where that provider does not work; the patient who was finally diagnosed and treated during incarceration may be unable to access care in the community.

Long-acting injectable (LAIs) medications can provide stability that survives these disruptions. The patient receiving monthly or bimonthly injections does not need to remember to take daily pills, does not need to maintain continuous access to a pharmacy, and maintains therapeutic drug levels even if they miss appointments or experience lapses in care. LAIs help lower the chances of relapse and rehospitalization in individuals with psychotic disorders. For some patients with severe bipolar disorder, LAI antipsychotics provide similar benefits. The choice to use an LAI should be made collaboratively, with the patient understanding both the benefits—stability, freedom from daily pills, reduced relapse—and the implications, including the commitment to regular injections and the inability to rapidly discontinue if side effects emerge.

Mistrust and Survival-Driven Nonadherence

Incarcerated and formerly incarcerated individuals often mistrust the systems that are supposed to help them, and this mistrust is frequently warranted. They may have been treated poorly by correctional healthcare providers, may have had medication used as a tool of control rather than care, may have experienced the healthcare system as an extension of the carceral system rather than as a separate realm governed by different values. This mistrust affects engagement with care after release; the patient may associate psychiatric treatment with incarceration itself and resist engagement as a form of resistance to the entire system.

Nonadherence in this population may reflect survival-driven decision-making rather than irrationality or illness. The patient who stops taking medication after release may be avoiding side effects that interfere with work, may be prioritizing other urgent needs like housing and food, may be avoiding the stigma of psychiatric medication in their community, or may be rejecting what feels like continued control by systems that have controlled them for too long. The clinician who approaches nonadherence with curiosity rather than judgment, who asks what is getting in the way and listens to the answer, is more likely to find solutions that work than the clinician who lectures about the importance of medication.

Harm Reduction and Dignity

Psychopharmacology in this population often leads to harm reduction. The goals may need to be realistic: not perfect symptom control but enough stability to avoid re-incarceration; not complete abstinence from substances but reduction in the most dangerous use; not a pristine treatment plan but engagement of any kind with care. The clinician must meet patients where they are, which may be far from where textbook treatment plans assume patients start.

Psychopharmacology in this population is also dignity restoration. Many incarcerated and formerly incarcerated individuals have been treated as less than human, their suffering dismissed, their needs ignored, their autonomy erased. The clinical encounter that treats them with respect, which asks about their preferences, which explains rather than dictates, which acknowledges their expertise on their own experience—this encounter may be itself therapeutic, independent of what medication is prescribed.

V. Immigrants, Refugees, and Cultural Context

Immigrants and refugees bring to the clinical encounter experiences, beliefs, and symptoms that may not fit easily into Western psychiatric categories. They may have survived war, persecution, torture, and displacement. They may have lost family members, homes, and entire ways of life. They may have made perilous journeys across deserts or seas, experienced detention, and uncertainty, and faced hostility and discrimination in their destination country. These experiences shape their psychiatric presentations in ways that require cultural humility and contextual understanding.

Somatic Idioms of Distress

Symptoms in immigrant and refugee populations often present somatically. The patient may come with complaints of headache, dizziness, chest pain, or abdominal distress rather than describing sadness, worry, or fear. This is not because they do not experience psychological distress but because the cultural idioms for expressing distress differ, because somatic symptoms may be less stigmatizing than psychiatric symptoms, or because the mind-body dualism that structures Western medicine does not map onto their understanding of illness.

The clinician who interprets somatic complaints at face value, ordering test after test in search of a medical explanation, will miss the underlying psychiatric condition. The clinician who dismisses somatic complaints as "just psychological" will invalidate the patient's suffering and lose their trust. The path forward requires holding both possibilities—that the symptoms are real and distressing, and that they may be manifestations of depression, anxiety, or trauma that can respond to psychiatric treatment.

Language and Communication

Language barriers complicate every aspect of care—history-taking, diagnosis, explanation of treatment, assessment of understanding, and detection of subtle symptoms. Working through interpreters is essential when patient and clinician do not share a language, but interpretation introduces its own complexities. The interpreter may soften or alter what the patient says, the patient may be uncomfortable discussing certain topics with the interpreter present, particularly if the interpreter is from their community; nuances of expression that would be diagnostically significant may be lost in translation.

When possible, professional interpreters trained in medical interpretation should be used rather than family members or ad hoc interpreters. Family members may have their own agendas, may be uncomfortable translating certain content, and may burden the patient with the knowledge that intimate disclosures are being shared with family. Children should never be used as interpreters for their parents' psychiatric care; the role reversal and exposure to adult content is inappropriate and potentially harmful.

Stigma and Help-Seeking

Mental illness carries different degrees and types of stigmas in different cultures. In some communities, psychiatric symptoms may be understood as spiritual affliction, as failure of character, or as shame upon the family. Seeking psychiatric treatment may be seen as an admission of weakness, as inappropriate airing of private matters, or as a betrayal of cultural values that emphasize family self-sufficiency. These beliefs affect whether patients seek care, what they disclose when they do, and whether they adhere to treatment.

The clinician must approach these cultural differences with humility rather than judgment, recognizing that Western psychiatric categories and treatments are not universal truths but one framework among many. This does not mean abandoning evidence-based treatment; it means offering treatment in ways that are culturally acceptable, explaining the rationale in terms that make sense within the patient's worldview, and respecting the patient's right to accept or decline treatment based on their own values.

Medication in Cultural Context

Medication requires careful explanation, particularly for patients unfamiliar with Western medicine or skeptical of psychiatric treatment. The clinician should explain what the medication is, how it works, what to expect, and what side effects might occur. Checking for understanding is essential—not just asking "do you understand?" but asking the patient to explain in their own words what they understood.

Medication response may differ across ethnic groups due to pharmacogenetic differences in drug metabolism, though the clinical significance of these differences is often modest. More important may be differences in medication-taking behavior, expectations about treatment, and interpretation of side effects. The patient from a culture that values stoic endurance may not report side effects; the patient from a culture that expects immediate relief may become discouraged and discontinue medication before it has had time to work; the patient who expects medicine to be natural may be uncomfortable with synthetic pharmaceuticals.

Diagnosis Requires Context

Diagnosis in immigrant and refugee populations cannot be separated from context. The patient who appears paranoid may be realistically fearful based on their experiences of persecution. The patient who appears depressed may be grieving losses that Western psychiatry does not fully comprehend. The patient who appears anxious may be responding rationally to uncertainty about immigration status, family safety, or economic survival. Pathologizing these responses—labeling as disorder what is actually reasonable reaction to extraordinary circumstances—does a disservice to patients and distorts diagnosis.

At the same time, immigrants and refugees do develop psychiatric disorders that require treatment. The challenge is to distinguish between the distress that is an expected response to their circum-stances and the distress that represents disorder superimposed on those circumstances. This distinction is not always clear, and in many cases, it may not matter for treatment purposes—treating the depres-sion or anxiety or PTSD may be appropriate regardless of how much of the patient's suffering is attributable to disorder versus circumstance.

VI. LGBTQ+ Populations

Individuals who are lesbian, gay, bisexual, transgender, queer, or who hold other sexual or gender minority identities experience elevated rates of depression, anxiety, suicidality, substance use, and trauma. These disparities do not reflect anything inherent to being LGBTQ+; they reflect the effects of minority stress—the chronic stress of living in a society that stigmatizes, discriminates against, and in some cases criminalizes or violently attacks minority identities.

Minority Stress and Its Consequences

Minority stress includes external stressors such as discrimination, harassment, and violence, as well as internal stressors such as inter-nalized stigma, expectations of rejection, and the need to conceal one's identity. These stressors are chronic, often beginning in child-hood or adolescence and continuing throughout life. Their cumula-tive effect produces the elevated psychiatric morbidity observed in LGBTQ+ populations.

The experience of rejection by family is particularly damaging. LGBTQ+ youth who experience family rejection have dramatically elevated rates of depression, substance use, and suicidality compared to those whose families are accepting. For many LGBTQ+ individu-als, family rejection is a formative trauma that shapes their relation-ship to intimacy, trust, and their own worth.

Religious condemnation adds another layer of harm to those raised in faith traditions that condemn their identities. The conflict between religious identity and sexual or gender identity can be profound, producing guilt, shame, and existential distress. Some individuals resolve this conflict by leaving their faith; others find or create affirming faith communities; still others remain caught in painful contradiction.

Clinical Implications

LGBTQ+ patients deserve clinicians who are knowledgeable about LGBTQ+ health, who use appropriate language, and who create clinical environments where patients feel safe to disclose their identities. This begins with intake forms that include options beyond male and female, which ask about sexual orientation rather than assuming heterosexuality, and that allow patients to specify their chosen name and pronouns. It continues with clinical interactions that do not assume the gender of partners, which normalize LGBTQ+ identities, and that demonstrate comfort with discussing sexuality and gender.

Affirmation itself is therapeutic. The clinician who responds to a patient's disclosure of LGBTQ+ identity with acceptance, with interest, with normalization communicates something that many LGBTQ+ patients have rarely experienced from authority figures. This acceptance does not cure psychiatric illness, but it creates the conditions in which treatment can be effective. The patient who must hide their identity from their clinician, who fears judgment or rejection, who experiences the clinical encounter as another site of minority stress, is unlikely to fully engage in treatment.

Medication Considerations

Medication selection in LGBTQ+ patients follows general principles, with attention to specific considerations relevant to this population. Sexual side effects of psychiatric medications may be particularly distressing for patients whose sexuality is already a site of complexity or conflict. Weight gain may be especially problematic for patients with body image concerns, which are elevated in some LGBTQ+ subpopulations. These concerns should be addressed proactively, with medication selection considering patient preferences and priorities.

For transgender patients receiving hormone therapy, potential interactions with psychiatric medications should be considered. Estrogen affects the metabolism of some medications, and testosterone may as well, though clinically significant interactions are not common. More important than pharmacokinetic interactions are the psychiatric impact of hormone therapy itself. For many transgender individuals, initiating hormone therapy produces profound improvements in mood, anxiety, and well-being—effects that may be more significant than any psychiatric medication. For others, the changes may bring unexpected complexity. The clinician should ask about hormone therapy, should understand its typical effects, and should consider its role in the patient's overall psychiatric picture.

VII. Clinical Illustrations from the Margins

A Veteran Whose Insomnia Reflected Unceasing Vigilance

A forty-three-year-old veteran presented with chronic insomnia that had persisted since his return from deployment eight years earlier. He had seen multiple providers, had tried multiple sleep medications, and had been told that his insomnia was due to poor sleep hygiene. He worked as a security guard, a job he chose because he could not tolerate the unpredictability of other work environments and because it gave structure to his hypervigilance, his constant scanning of the environment, his positioning to see doors and exits, his inability to relax in public spaces.

His insomnia was not a sleep disorder; it was a trauma response. His nervous system had learned in combat that letting down one's guard could mean death. That learning had not unlearned itself when he returned home. Every night, as he tried to fall asleep, his body resisted the vulnerability of unconsciousness. His ears remained alert for sounds; his muscles remained tensed for action; his mind remained scanning for threat. No sleep hygiene intervention could override this neurobiological vigilance.

Treatment began with recognition of what his symptoms meant —that his insomnia was not weakness or failure but the continued operation of survival mechanisms that had kept him alive in war. Prazosin reduced his nightmares and the dread that accompanied bedtime. An SSRI reduced his overall level of arousal. Therapy focused on gradually teaching his nervous system that safety was possible—not through reassurance, which his mind dismissed, but through the slow accumulation of experiences in which he was vulnerable and nothing bad happened.

His sleep improved, though it never became easy. More importantly, he understood himself differently. He was not broken; he was adapted to a world that no longer existed. Treatment was the slow process of adaptation to a new world-a process that required patience, which honored what he had survived, and that did not demand that he simply decide to feel safe.

An Autistic Woman Misdiagnosed with Anxiety for Decades

A fifty-two-year-old woman came for a second opinion after decades of treatment for anxiety that had never quite worked. She had been on and off various SSRIs, had tried buspirone and gabapentin, had engaged in cognitive-behavioral therapy focused on catastrophic thinking and avoidance. She described her anxiety as constant-a background hum of overwhelm that intensified in social situations, in unpredictable environments, in any setting where she could not control the stimuli.

She had always been "different," she said, though she had learned to hide it. As a child, she preferred books to playmates, had intense interests that other children found strange, and was over- whelmed by the noise of the cafeteria and the chaos of the play- ground. As an adult, she had learned the rules of social interaction through conscious study, but social events remained exhausting, requiring enormous effort to appear normal. She had developed routines that structured her life and became distressed when those routines were disrupted. She experienced fabrics, sounds, and lights that others found unremarkable as intensely, sometimes painfully, stimulating.

The diagnosis was autism spectrum disorder, not generalized anxiety disorder. Her "anxiety" was largely autistic distress—the over- whelm of a nervous system that processed sensory information differently, the exhaustion of masking her natural way of being to meet neurotypical expectations, the distress that arose when predictability was lost. Her anxiety treatments had failed because they were treating the wrong condition.

The diagnosis was itself therapeutic. She finally had a framework for understanding her lifelong experience of difference, her exhaus- tion, her need for routines and predictability, her difficulty with small talk and her depth with special interests. She was not anxious; she was autistic. She was not failing at being normal; she was succeeding at an impossibly difficult masquerade.

Treatment shifted. Accommodations became more important than medication—reducing sensory demands, protecting time for recovery after social exertion, giving herself permission to stop masking when she could. A low dose of an SSRI helped with the residual anxiety; noise-canceling headphones helped more. The goal was not to make her neurotypical but to make her life sustainable as an autistic person in a neurotypical world.

A Refugee Whose Depression Spoke Through Pain

A sixty-year-old man who had fled persecution in his home country presented with chronic pain—headaches, back pain, abdominal pain—that had been evaluated repeatedly without finding a cause. He had been told his pain was "stress-related," a formulation he found dismissive and insulting. He did not trust doctors; he experienced medical encounters as interrogations in which he was suspected of malingering or exaggerating.

His history, when it finally emerged, explained everything. He had been imprisoned and tortured for his political beliefs before fleeing his country. He had lost his brother in that prison. He had spent years in refugee camps before arriving in the United States, where he was an educated man reduced to menial work, separated from everything familiar, struggling with a language he had never fully mastered.

He did not use the word "depression." In his cultural framework, physical pain was acceptable—a man could have pain—while psychological suffering was shameful. His pain was real; the question was not whether his symptoms were genuine but how to understand them. In his case, the pain was a somatic expression of psychological anguish, the body speaking what the mind could not say, the trauma, loss, and displacement manifesting in the flesh.

Treatment required patience. He needed to believe that his pain was taken seriously before he could consider that it might have psychological dimensions. An antidepressant that also addressed pain—duloxetine—was framed as treatment for his chronic pain, which it genuinely was. Slowly, as his pain improved, he became willing to talk about what had happened to him—not in terms of mental illness but in terms of his story, his losses, his survival. He never accepted that he was depressed, but he did accept that what he had been through had affected his body, and he did accept treatment that helped.

VIII. Prescribing at the Margins

In special populations, there is no neutral prescribing. Every medication decision occurs within a context of power, history, and meaning that shapes how the prescription is experienced and whether it helps or harms.

Context-Aware Practice

The clinician treating special populations must understand the contexts in which patients live—not as background information but as central to diagnosis and treatment. The homeless patient cannot maintain medication requiring refrigeration; the patient with food insecurity cannot take medication that must be taken with food; the patient fleeing domestic violence cannot safely keep medication where an abuser might find it. These practical realities shape what is possible and must be integrated into treatment planning.

Context also includes the social determinants that shape health: poverty, discrimination, housing instability, food insecurity, exposure to violence, and lack of access to care. Medication that is effective in clinical trials may fail in practice if patients cannot fill prescriptions, cannot afford copays, cannot get to appointments, or cannot prioritize medication when they are struggling to survive. Effective treatment in these populations requires addressing these barriers, whether through patient assistance programs, transportation support, flexible scheduling, or advocacy for patients' broader needs.

Trauma-Informed Practice

Trauma-informed care recognizes that trauma is common, that it shapes how patients experience medical encounters, and that the clinical interaction itself can be retraumatizing or healing depending on how it is conducted. The trauma-informed clinician does not require disclosure of trauma history; they assume that many patients carry such histories and conduct themselves accordingly. They prioritize safety, predictability, and patient control. They explain what they are doing and why. They ask permission before physical examinations. They respond to distress with curiosity rather than judgment.

In prescribing, trauma-informed practice means attending to how medications might replicate or counteract traumatic dynamics. Medications that produce sedation, cognitive dulling, or a sense of being controlled may be particularly distressing to trauma survivors. Medications that restore agency, which are chosen collaboratively, that are explained transparently are more likely to be accepted and used effectively.

Ethically Grounded Practice

Prescribing in special populations raises ethical questions that do not arise in the same way with more privileged patients. When a patient refuses treatment that would clearly help them, is this autonomous choice to be respected or illness impairing judgment to be overridden? When a patient is nonadherent- is this a problem to be solved or a communication to be understood? When a patient from a marginalized community mistrusts the medical establishment, is this pathological suspicion or reasonable self-protection?

These questions do not have easy answers, but they require that the clinician approach them with ethical seriousness rather than defaulting to what is easiest. The values that should guide practice— respect for autonomy, commitment to benefit, obligation to avoid harm, attention to justice—must be actively applied to each situation rather than assumed to resolve it.

Humility and Learning

Finally, prescribing in special populations requires humility. The clinician will not always know what is right. They will not fully understand experiences they themselves have not experienced. They will make mistakes, will miss things, or will fail patients despite their best intentions. This is not cause for paralysis but for ongoing learning—from patients, from colleagues, from literature, from reflection on what has worked and what has not.

The patients at the margins have much to teach if the clinician is willing to learn. Their survival strategies, their critiques of systems that have failed them, their knowledge of their own experience-these are resources for better care. The clinician who approaches these patients as experts on their own lives, who listens before prescribing, who remains curious about what they do not yet understand, will provide better care than the clinician who assumes they already know what these patients need.

IX. Conclusion

Special populations remind us that psychiatry occurs in the world —not in the controlled conditions of clinical trials but in lives shaped by trauma, difference, discrimination, displacement, and disadvantage. Medication is one tool among many, and it cannot be separated from the contexts in which it is prescribed and taken.

Wisdom in treating these populations lies in seeing what is not obvious- the trauma behind irritability, the autism behind the anxiety, the cultural framework that shapes symptom expression, the survival logic that underlies apparent nonadherence. It lies in offering treatment that respects autonomy, which acknowledges history, which adapts to context, and that honors the resilience that has allowed patients to survive what they have survived.

The clinician who treats special populations will often feel uncertain, will often lack clear guidelines, will often have to improvise and adapt. This is not a sign of failure; it is the nature of the work. The patients at the margins require more of us-more humility, more flexibility, more willingness to question our assumptions and learn from our mistakes.

What we offer in return is the possibility of treatment that reaches patients who have been passed up by standard approaches, that meets them where they are rather than where textbooks assume they should be, and that contributes to healing in contexts where healing has been hard to find.

~

12

WHEN THE IMMUNE SYSTEM ATTACKS THE MIND

PANDAS, PANS, AND THE NEW FRONTIER OF PSYCHOIMMUNOLOGY

The Child Who Changed Overnight

I magine tucking your cheerful, confident eight-year-old into bed one evening, only to wake the next morning to a child you barely recognize. Overnight, she has become terrified of contamination, washing her hands until they bleed. She screams that she cannot swallow her breakfast, convinced she will choke. She blinks and grimaces in strange, repetitive patterns. When you try to comfort her, she flies into a rage so intensely it frightens you both. The pediatrician finds nothing wrong. The school psychologist suggests anxiety. But you know—with the certainty only a parent possesses—that something has hijacked your daughter's brain.

This scenario, once dismissed as impossible or exaggerated, now has a name and a scientific explanation. We are living through a revolution in our understanding of mental illness, one that reveals an astonishing truth: sometimes the immune system, that vigilant defender against infection, turns traitor and attacks the very brain it was designed to protect. The result is psychiatric illness that appears suddenly, progresses rapidly, and—most remarkably—may be treated not with traditional psychiatric medications alone, but with approaches borrowed from immunology and infectious disease medicine.

This chapter explores PANDAS, PANS, and related psycho-immunological conditions across the entire human lifespan. We will examine how these disorders are diagnosed, what other conditions accompany them, and how they are treated. Most importantly, we will glimpse a future in which the artificial boundary between phys-ical and mental illness finally dissolves, opening new therapeutic possibilities that would have seemed like science fiction just a genera-tion ago.

A Brief History of Mind-Body Medicine

The idea that infections could cause psychiatric symptoms is not new, though it has traveled a long and winding road to acceptance. In the late nineteenth and early twentieth centuries, physicians observed that patients recovering from influenza, scarlet fever, or rheumatic fever sometimes developed unusual neurological and psychiatric symptoms. The great encephalitis lethargica epidemic of 1917 to 1928, which followed the devastating Spanish flu pandemic, left thousands of survivors with profound neuropsychiatric changes —parkinsonism, catatonia, and personality alterations that could persist for decades.

Rheumatic fever, caused by group A streptococcal infection, provided particularly compelling evidence. Physicians had long noted that some children with rheumatic fever developed Sydenham chorea, a movement disorder characterized by involuntary jerking and writhing. They also observed that these children frequently experienced emotional changes: tearfulness, irritability, obsessive thoughts, and difficulty concentrating. The connection seemed obvi-ous-the same streptococcal infection that could damage heart valves was somehow affecting the brain.

Yet as the twentieth century progressed and psychiatry increas-ingly separated from general medicine, these observations faded from mainstream awareness. The Freudian revolution emphasized psychological causation. The biological psychiatry movement that followed focused on neurotransmitter imbalances. Neither frame-work had much room for the immune system.

The tide began to turn in 1998, when Dr. Susan Swedo and her colleagues at the National Institute of Mental Health published a landmark paper describing a subset of children who developed sudden-onset obsessive-compulsive disorder and tic disorders following streptococcal infections. They named this condition Pedi-atric Autoimmune Neuropsychiatric Disorders Associated with Streptococcal Infections, or PANDAS. The paper ignited fierce controversy that continues to this day, but it also launched a new field of inquiry that has fundamentally changed how we think about at least some psychiatric illness.

UNDERSTANDING AUTOIMMUNITY: **When Defense Becomes Attack**

To comprehend PANDAS, PANS, and related conditions, we must first understand autoimmunity. The immune system faces an extraor-dinarily difficult task: it must recognize and destroy an almost infinite variety of foreign invaders while leaving the body's own tissues unharmed. This discrimination between self and non-self is accom-plished through an elaborate system of checks and balances devel-oped over millions of years of evolution.

Antibodies are proteins produced by immune cells that recognize specific molecular patterns on invaders. When bacteria or viruses enter the body, the immune system generates antibodies that bind to proteins on the invader's surface, marking it for destruction. This system works remarkably well most of the time.

Problems arise when the molecular patterns on an invader happen to resemble patterns on the body's own tissues—a phenomenon called molecular mimicry. In this situation, antibodies designed to attack the invader may also attack the body's own cells. The immune system, unable to distinguish friend from foe, turns its formidable weapons inward.

In rheumatic fever, antibodies directed against group A strepto-coccal bacteria cross-react with proteins in the heart, joints, and brain. The result is inflammation and damage to these organs—even after the original bacterial infection has been cleared. The bacteria are long gone, but the immune response they triggered continues its assault.

The brain presents a special case. For many years, scientists believed the brain was "immune privileged," meaning largely isolated from the immune system by the blood-brain barrier. We now know this is an oversimplification. Immune cells can and do enter the brain under certain circumstances. Antibodies can cross the blood-brain barrier, especially when this barrier has been made more permeable by inflammation. Immune signaling molecules called cytokines, produced throughout the body during infection and inflammation, profoundly affect brain function even without entering the brain directly.

When autoimmune processes target the brain, the results can be devastating. Depending on which brain regions are affected, patients may experience movement disorders, seizures, cognitive impair-ment, psychosis, depression, anxiety, obsessive-compulsive symp-toms, or personality changes. Often multiple symptoms occur together, reflecting widespread inflammation across different brain networks.

PANDAS: The Condition That Started It All

PANDAS remains the most studied and most controversial of psycho-immunological disorders. The diagnostic criteria, refined over more than two decades, include five essential elements.

First, the patient must have obsessive-compulsive disorder or a tic disorder, or both. The obsessive-compulsive symptoms in PANDAS often differ from typical childhood OCD. Contamination fears and washing compulsions are common, but so are unusual concerns about symmetry, fears of harm coming to loved ones, and intrusive violent or sexual thoughts that horrify the child experiencing them. Tics may be simple, like eye blinking or throat clearing, or complex, involving sequences of movements or vocalizations.

Second, symptom onset must be prepubertal. PANDAS, by definition, begins before puberty, typically between ages three and twelve. This age restriction likely reflects developmental changes in immune function and blood-brain barrier permeability that occur with puberty.

Third, symptom onset must be acute and dramatic. This is perhaps the most distinctive feature of PANDAS. Rather than the gradual worsening typically seen in childhood OCD or Tourette syndrome, PANDAS begins suddenly—often described by parents as occurring overnight or within a few days. A child who showed no previous psychiatric symptoms develops severe, impairing symptoms essentially without warning.

Fourth, there must be a temporal relationship to group A streptococcal infection. Symptoms begin shortly after a streptococcal infection, such as strep throat or scarlet fever, and may worsen with subsequent infections. This temporal association is the key to the "associated with streptococcal infections" in the PANDAS name. It does not mean every strep infection will cause a flare; nor will the symptoms appear immediately upon infection. The relationship is probabilistic rather than deterministic.

Fifth, the patient must have associated neurological abnormalities. These may include choreiform movements (subtle, irregular movements visible when the child extends the arms and spreads the fingers), deterioration in handwriting, or other neurological signs. Some children develop urinary frequency or nighttime urinary accidents. Sleep disturbances are nearly universal.

Beyond these core criteria, PANDAS is typically accompanied by a constellation of associated features. Separation anxiety often becomes severe, with children unable to leave their parents' side or on the other hand refusing to attend school. Irritability and emotional lability are common, with children experiencing dramatic mood swings or becoming uncharacteristically aggressive. Many children develop restricted eating, sometimes severe enough to require hospitalization. Cognitive changes are frequently reported, including difficulty with concentration, memory problems, and a decline in academic performance. Some children become unusually sensitive to sensory stimuli—textures of clothing, sounds, or lights that never bothered them before becoming intolerable.

The diagnosis of PANDAS remains clinical; there is no laboratory test that definitively confirms or excludes the condition. Evidence of recent streptococcal infection supports the diagnosis but is not always obtainable, as antibodies may not yet have risen or may have already fallen by the time the child is evaluated. Throat cultures may be negative if the infection has been resolved. Some children are streptococcal carriers who harbor the bacteria without active infection, complicating interpretation.

The lack of a definitive diagnostic test, combined with the dramatic nature of the proposed mechanism and the limitations of early research, fueled skepticism that persists in some quarters today. Critics argued that the apparent association between streptococcal infection and psychiatric symptoms could be coincidental, given how common both are in childhood. They noted that the original studies were small and potentially subject to selection bias. They worried that accepting PANDAS would lead to inappropriate antibiotic use and distraction from proven psychiatric treatments.

Proponents countered with growing evidence from larger studies, biological plausibility based on the established precedent of Sydenham Chorea, and the testimony of countless families whose observations could not be dismissed as mere coincidence. The debate grew acrimonious at times, with implications for children caught in the middle—some receiving treatments that genuinely helped them, others denied intervention by skeptical providers, still others subjected to unnecessary or potentially harmful treatments by well-meaning but overeager clinicians.

Today, the consensus has shifted toward acceptance that PANDAS represents a real clinical entity, though questions remain about its precise boundaries, underlying mechanisms, and optimal treatment. Research continues to refine our understanding, but few serious scientists now deny that poststreptococcal autoimmune brain inflammation can cause or exacerbate psychiatric symptoms in at least some children.

PANS: Broadening the Concept

As researchers studied PANDAS, they encountered a puzzle. Some children presented with the same dramatic, sudden-onset symptoms and clinical picture but without evidence of streptococcal infection. Their symptoms seemed to follow other infections—influenza, mycoplasma pneumonia, Epstein-Barr virus, Lyme disease —or occurred without any identifiable infectious trigger at all. The PANDAS framework, tied specifically to streptococcal infection, could not accommodate these cases.

In 2012, a consortium of researchers proposed a broader diagnostic category: Pediatric Acute-onset Neuropsychiatric Syndrome, or PANS. The PANS criteria preserved the essential feature of abrupt onset while removing the requirement for streptococcal association.

PANS defined by three criteria- First, there must be abrupt, dramatic onset of obsessive-compulsive disorder or severely restricted food intake. The acute onset remains central feature-symptoms appear suddenly rather than developing gradually over weeks or months. Second, the psychiatric symptoms must be accompanied by at least two of the following: anxiety, emotional lability or depression, irritability or aggression, behavioral regression, deterioration in school performance, sensory or motor abnormalities, or somatic signs including sleep disturbances and urinary symptoms. Third, symptoms must not be better explained by a known neurological or medical disorder.

PANS serves as an overarching classification that includes PANDAS (specifically associated with streptococcal infections) as well as analogous clinical presentations resulting from other infectious agents, metabolic abnormalities, or unidentified causes. This broader framework acknowledges that autoimmune brain inflammation can arise through multiple pathways, not all of which involve streptococcal bacteria.

The PANS formulation has proven clinically useful, providing a diagnostic home for children whose presentations strongly suggest immune-mediated brain dysfunction even when no streptococcal trigger can be identified. It has also encouraged research into other potential triggers and mechanisms, enriching our understanding of the complex relationships between infection, immunity, and brain function.

BEYOND CHILDHOOD: **Psychoimmunology Across the Lifespan**

PANDAS and PANS were initially described in children, and the prepubertal onset requirement remains part of the PANDAS definition. However, the underlying mechanisms—molecular mimicry, autoantibody formation, neuroinflammation—have no inherent age limit. This has led researchers and clinicians to ask: what happens to children with PANDAS or PANS as they grow up, and can similar processes cause psychiatric illness in adolescents and adults?

The answers emerging from research suggest that psycho-immunological disorders are indeed not limited to childhood, though they may manifest differently across the lifespan.

Some children with PANDAS or PANS continue to experience symptoms progressing into adolescence and adulthood. For some, the condition burns out, and they recover fully with or without treatment. Others experience persistent or relapsing symptoms that evolve over time. A child whose primary symptom was obsessive-compulsive disorder may develop depression or anxiety as predominant features in adolescence. The dramatic episodic flares triggered by infection may give way to more chronic, fluctuating symptoms. Whether this represents evolution of the underlying autoimmune process, accumulated neural damage, or psychological adaptation to chronic illness remains unclear.

Perhaps more provocatively, researchers have begun identifying autoimmune mechanisms in psychiatric illnesses that first appear in adolescence or adulthood, raising the question of whether some proportion of adult mental illness has an unrecognized autoimmune component.

Autoimmune encephalitis, particularly anti-NMDA receptor encephalitis, provides the clearest example. This condition, first described in 2007, typically affects young adults, especially women. It often begins with psychiatric symptoms—psychosis, personality changes, agitation, hallucinations—that may initially be misdiagnosed as schizophrenia, bipolar disorder, or another primary psychiatric illness. Over days to weeks, patients develop seizures, movement abnormalities, autonomic instability, and decreased consciousness. Without treatment, the condition is often fatal. With immunotherapy, however, many patients recover substantially or completely.

Anti-NMDA receptor encephalitis is caused by antibodies that bind to NMDA receptors, critical components of the brain's glutamate signaling system. These receptors are essential for learning, memory, and cognitive flexibility. When antibodies interfere with their function, the result is a devastating neuropsychiatric syndrome. About half of cases are associated with tumors—typically ovarian teratomas in young women—that trigger antibody production. The other half occurs without any identifiable tumor, suggesting that infection or other immune triggers may be responsible.

The discovery of anti-NMDA receptor encephalitis has prompted reevaluation of psychiatric diagnoses across the board. Studies have found that a small but significant proportion of patients diagnosed with first-episode psychosis have detectable autoantibodies that may be contributing to their symptoms. The implications are profound: if even a minority of patients with schizophrenia, bipolar disorder, or severe depression have an autoimmune component to their illness, identifying and treating that component could fundamentally change their outcomes.

Other autoantibodies affecting brain function continue to be discovered. Antibodies to GABA receptors, glycine receptors, dopamine receptors, and various neuronal surface proteins have all been linked to neuropsychiatric syndromes. The clinical pictures vary depending on which proteins are targeted and which brain regions are most affected, but the common thread is psychiatric symptoms arising from immune attack on the brain.

Systemic autoimmune diseases—lupus, rheumatoid arthritis, Sjögren syndrome, and others—frequently have neuropsychiatric manifestations that may precede, accompany, or follow the more typical features of these conditions. Neuropsychiatric lupus, in particular, can present with psychosis, mood disorders, cognitive dysfunction, or seizures, sometimes without prominent systemic symptoms. The boundary between "psychiatric" and "medical" illness blurs to the point of meaninglessness in these cases.

Even in the absence of formal autoimmune disease, chronic low-grade inflammation has been linked to depression and other psychiatric conditions. Studies consistently find elevated inflammatory markers in subsets of depressed patients, and anti-inflammatory treatments show promise for some who have not responded to standard antidepressants. Whether this inflammation represents a cause, consequence, or correlate of depression remains an active area of investigation, but the relationship itself seems well established.

Aging brings its own immune changes that may affect brain function. The aging immune system tends toward increased inflammation —a phenomenon sometimes called "inflammaging"—while simultaneously becoming less effective at targeting specific threats. These changes may contribute to the cognitive decline and mood changes common in older adults. The relationship between immune function and dementia, including Alzheimer disease, is an area of intense current research, with some evidence suggesting that inflammatory processes contribute to neurodegeneration.

The emerging picture is one of continuous interaction between immune and nervous systems throughout life, with perturbations in this interaction potentially contributing to psychiatric illness at any age. The child with PANDAS and the elderly person with late-onset depression may have more in common than we ever suspected.

EVALUATION AND DIAGNOSIS: **Finding the Immune Fingerprint**

Diagnosing psycho-immunological disorders requires integrating clinical observation, laboratory testing, and often a degree of clinical judgment that makes some practitioners uncomfortable. There is no single test that definitively confirms PANDAS, PANS, or most other psycho-immunological conditions. Instead, diagnosis relies on recognizing characteristic patterns and systematically evaluating for immune involvement.

The clinical history is paramount. The sudden, dramatic onset that characterizes PANDAS and PANS immediately distinguishes these conditions from the more gradual development typical of most psychiatric disorders. Parents often describe their child as being "like a different person" or say the change happened "overnight." This history should prompt consideration of an immune-mediated process, particularly if symptoms began shortly after an infection.

A detailed infection history is essential. This includes not only obvious symptomatic infections but also possible exposures, family members with streptococcal infections, and any pattern of symptom worsening around infections. Children with PANDAS may not always be symptomatic during the triggering streptococcal infection—they may be carriers who harbor the bacteria without sore throat or fever, or they may have had such mild symptoms that the infection went unnoticed.

Physical and neurological examination may reveal subtle abnormalities. Choreiform movements, visible as irregular twitches, or jerks when the child extends the arms and spreads the fingers, support the diagnosis. Dilated pupils, decreased reflexes, or subtle motor coordination problems may be present. The examination should also assess for signs of systemic illness that might suggest other autoimmune or inflammatory conditions.

Laboratory testing serves several purposes: documenting evidence of recent infection, assessing for inflammation, and in some cases detecting specific autoantibodies.

Streptococcal testing includes throat culture, rapid streptococcal antigen test, and blood tests for streptococcal antibodies. The anti-streptolysin O (ASO) and anti-DNase B titers rise after streptococcal infection and may remain elevated for weeks to months. A single elevated titer suggests recent infection, but rising titers over time provide stronger evidence. However, titers may be normal if measured too early (before the immune response develops) or too late (after titers have declined). Normal titers do not exclude PANDAS, and elevated titers in an area where streptococcal infection is common may not be specific.

Inflammatory markers such as erythrocyte sedimentation rate and C-reactive protein may be elevated during acute flares but are often normal, particularly between episodes. Their normalcy does not exclude immune-mediated disease.

Testing for other infections may be warranted depending on the clinical picture. Mycoplasma pneumonia, Epstein-Barr virus, cytomegalovirus, Lyme disease, and influenza have all been associated with PANS-like presentations. The choice of testing should be guided by symptoms, exposure history, and regional prevalence of various infections.

Autoantibody testing is evolving. Several commercial panels claim to detect antibodies associated with PANDAS and PANS, but their clinical utility remains controversial. The best-validated autoantibodies are those associated with autoimmune encephalitis—anti-NMDA receptor antibodies and related antibodies detectable in blood and cerebrospinal fluid. When autoimmune encephalitis is suspected based on clinical features such as seizures, severe cognitive impairment, or movement abnormalities beyond simple tics, testing for these antibodies is essential and well-supported by evidence.

Brain imaging is typically normal in PANDAS and PANS, though research studies have identified subtle abnormalities in brain volume and function. Imaging is most useful for excluding other conditions that might explain the symptoms. In cases of suspected autoimmune encephalitis, magnetic resonance imaging may show characteristic abnormalities, particularly in the temporal lobes.

Lumbar puncture to analyze cerebrospinal fluid is indicated when autoimmune encephalitis is suspected or when the clinical picture is severe or atypical. Findings may include elevated white blood cells, elevated protein, or the presence of specific autoantibodies. Normal cerebrospinal fluid does not exclude immune-mediated brain disease but makes some diagnoses less likely.

The diagnostic process should also assess to rule out conditions that commonly co-occur with or mimic psycho-immunological disorders. Thyroid function should be checked, as autoimmune thyroid disease can cause psychiatric symptoms and often co-occurs with other autoimmune conditions. Assessment looking for other autoimmune diseases may be warranted based on symptoms and family history.

Ultimately, diagnosis often requires synthesizing imperfect information to form a clinical judgment. A child with sudden-onset OCD and tics following a documented streptococcal infection presents a relatively clear picture. A teenager with gradual-onset depression and no clear infection history but a family history of autoimmune disease and a few subtle inflammatory markers present a much more ambiguous case. Clinicians must weigh the evidence, consider the potential benefits and risks of various treatment approaches, and often make decisions under uncertainty.

This ambiguity troubles some clinicians accustomed to more definitive diagnostic categories. However, uncertainty is inherent in medicine, and the alternative—ignoring the possibility of immune-mediated illness because it cannot be definitively proven—means condemning some patients to inadequate treatment. The key is to maintain appropriate humility about what we do and do not know, to remain open to revising assessments as new information emerges, and to proceed thoughtfully with treatment while monitoring carefully for response.

Comorbidities: The Company These Conditions Keep

Psycho-immunological disorders rarely occur in isolation. Understanding the conditions that frequently accompany them is essential for comprehensive evaluation and treatment.

Anxiety disorders are nearly universal in PANDAS and PANS. Separation anxiety, in which the child becomes extremely distressed when separated from parents, is particularly common and often severe. Generalized anxiety, social anxiety, and panic symptoms also occur. The anxiety often has an existential quality—children may express fears of death, of their parents dying, or of impending catastrophe—that seems more typically associated with adult anxiety than childhood worries.

Mood disturbances are common, including depressive symptoms and marked emotional lability. Children may cry inconsolably one moment and rage the next, with little apparent provocation. This emotional instability often exhausts and confuses parents, who may be accused of spoiling or mismanaging their child when in reality the child's nervous system is simply dysregulated.

Attention and cognitive problems frequently accompany PANDAS and PANS. Parents and teachers notice that the child cannot concentrate, forgets things that were previously well learned, and seems mentally foggy. Academic performance typically declines. Standardized testing may reveal deficits in processing speed, working memory, or executive function. These cognitive symptoms, though less dramatic than the OCD or tics, can be among the most disabling aspects of the condition.

Sleep disturbances are extremely common. Insomnia, night-mares, night terrors, and disrupted sleep architecture all occur. Some children develop fear of sleeping alone that they did not have before illness onset. Others sleep excessively, particularly during acute flares. The relationship between sleep and immune function is bidi-rectional—immune activation disrupts sleep, and sleep deprivation impairs immune function—creating a potentially vicious cycle.

Eating disturbances range from decreased appetite during acute illness to severe restriction that resemble anorexia nervosa. Some children develop fear of swallowing, convinced that they will choke or that food is contaminated. Others become extremely selective about food textures, temperatures, or colors. These eating distur-bances can lead to significant weight loss and nutritional deficiencies if not addressed.

Urinary symptoms, particularly increased frequency, and bedwet-ting in previously toilet-trained children, occur commonly enough to be included in diagnostic criteria. The mechanism is not fully under-stood but may relate to inflammation affecting the autonomic nervous system.

Sensory sensitivities frequently emerge or worsen with illness onset. Children may find the tags in their clothing intolerable, cover their ears at normal sounds, or become distressed by ordinary lighting. These sensitivities resemble those seen in autism spectrum disorder, and indeed some children with PANDAS or PANS may meet criteria for autism spectrum disorder during acute episodes, even if they showed no such features before illness onset.

Motor symptoms beyond tics may include deterioration in handwriting, new clumsiness, or coordination problems, and the choreiform movements that are part of the diagnostic criteria. Some children develop frank Chorea similar to that seen in Sydenham Chorea.

Other autoimmune conditions occur at elevated rates in children with PANDAS and PANS and in their family members. Thyroid autoimmunity, rheumatoid arthritis, lupus, and celiac disease are all overrepresented. This clustering of autoimmune conditions suggests shared genetic susceptibility and should prompt clinicians to consider and screen for related conditions.

Primary psychiatric disorders may coexist with psycho-immunological disorders, either predating them or emerging independently. A child may have preexisting ADHD that worsens during PANDAS flares or may develop depression in adolescence that is genuinely separate from their earlier PANDAS. Distinguishing between ongoing immune-mediated symptoms and comorbid primary psychiatric illness is clinically challenging but important for guiding treatment.

TREATMENT: **A Multimodal Approach**

Treating psycho-immunological disorders requires a comprehensive approach that addresses both the immune dysfunction and the resulting neuropsychiatric symptoms. The optimal treatment strategy depends on the severity of symptoms, the clarity of the diagnosis, and the response to initial interventions.

Treatment can be conceptualized as occurring in three domains: addressing acute infection, modulating the immune response, and managing psychiatric symptoms. Most patients benefit from interventions across all three domains, though the relative emphasis varies depending on the clinical situation.

When active streptococcal infection is present, antibiotic treatment is straightforward and uncontroversial. Penicillin or amoxicillin remain first-line treatments for streptococcal pharyngitis, with alternatives available for penicillin-allergic patients. Treating acute infection may lead to improvement in psychiatric symptoms, though response is neither immediate nor guaranteed.

More controversial is the use of prophylactic antibiotics— ongoing antibiotic treatment intended to prevent future streptococcal infections and thereby prevent symptom flares. Several small studies have suggested benefit from prophylactic antibiotics in carefully selected patients with clear infection-triggered symptom patterns. The rationale is straightforward: if symptoms are triggered by streptococcal infection, preventing infection should prevent flares. However, concerns about antibiotic resistance, side effects, and the potential for overtreatment have limited widespread adoption of this approach. Current guidelines suggest considering prophylactic antibiotics for patients with clear temporal association between streptococcal infection and symptom exacerbation, but this remains an area of ongoing research and clinical judgment.

Immunomodulatory treatments aim to dampen the abnormal immune response that is causing brain inflammation. The intensity of immunomodulation typically correlates with symptom severity.

For mild to moderate cases, first-line anti-inflammatory treatment often includes nonsteroidal anti-inflammatory drugs such as ibuprofen or naproxen. Though typically thought of as pain relievers, these medications reduce inflammation throughout the body, including potentially in the brain. Some families report significant improvement with consistent anti-inflammatory medication, though controlled trials are limited.

Corticosteroids provide more potent anti-inflammatory effects and are sometimes used for acute flares or when other anti-inflammatory treatments prove insufficient. Short courses of oral prednisone or similar medications can produce dramatic improvement in some patients. However, the side effects of corticosteroids limit their long-term use, and symptoms may recur when the medication is stopped.

For moderate to severe cases that do not respond adequately to anti-inflammatory medications, more intensive immunomodulatory treatments may be considered.

Intravenous immunoglobulin, or IVIG, involves infusion of pooled antibodies from thousands of blood donors. IVIG modulates immune function through several mechanisms that are not fully understood, including providing blocking antibodies, affecting immune signaling, and altering antibody production. Multiple small trials have suggested benefit in PANDAS and PANS, and IVIG is now used fairly widely in specialty centers, though it remains expensive, requires intravenous access, and is not universally available. Side effects include headache, flu-like symptoms, and rarely more serious reactions.

Plasmapheresis, also called therapeutic plasma exchange, physically removes circulating antibodies by filtering the patient's blood. Studies in PANDAS have shown significant benefit from plasmapheresis, particularly for severe cases. However, the procedure is invasive, requires specialized facilities, and carries risks including infection and bleeding. It is typically reserved for severe cases that have not responded to other treatments.

Rituximab, a medication that depletes B cells (the immune cells that produce antibodies), has been used in refractory cases of autoimmune encephalitis and is sometimes considered for severe PANS. As an immunosuppressive medication, it carries significant risks and requires careful monitoring. Its use in PANS remains experimental.

Emerging immunomodulatory approaches continue to be investigated. Medications that target specific inflammatory pathways, rather than broadly suppressing immune function, hold promise for more targeted treatment with fewer side effects. However, most remain in early stages of research for psycho-immunological disorders.

While addressing the immune aspects of illness is essential, most patients also benefit from psychiatric treatments aimed at managing symptoms and supporting recovery.

Cognitive behavioral therapy remains the gold standard psychological treatment for obsessive-compulsive disorder, including OCD associated with PANDAS and PANS. The core technique, exposure and response prevention, involves gradually confronting feared situations while resisting compulsive behaviors. For children with PANDAS and PANS, therapy may need to be modified based on symptom severity and the child's cognitive state. During acute severe flares, intensive exposure therapy may not be feasible or appropriate; simpler supportive approaches may be more helpful until the child stabilizes. As symptoms improve, more active engagement with exposure-based treatment becomes possible.

Family therapy and parent training are essential components of treatment. Parents need to understand the nature of the illness, learn strategies for responding to symptoms without inadvertently reinforcing them, and receive support for the enormous stress of caring for a child with sudden-onset psychiatric illness. Family accommodation-the well-intentioned adjustments families make to work around a child's symptoms—can sometimes perpetuate symptoms and should be addressed thoughtfully.

School accommodations are often necessary during acute illness and recovery. Depending on symptom severity, accommodations may range from extended time on tests and reduced homework to home tutoring or temporary medical leave. The goal is to maintain educational progress while avoiding overwhelming a child whose cognitive resources are already strained.

Psychiatric medications have an important role in symptom management, though their use in PANDAS and PANS requires some nuance. The medications typically used for OCD and tics—serotonin reuptake inhibitors and antipsychotics—are often helpful, but some children with PANDAS and PANS seem unusually sensitive to these medications, experiencing significant side effects at doses that would typically be well tolerated. Starting at low doses and increasing slowly is advisable. Some clinicians observe that psychiatric medications become more effective after immunomodulatory treatment has reduced underlying inflammation, suggesting that addressing the immune component may enhance response to standard psychiatric approaches.

Serotonin reuptake inhibitors remain first-line medication treatment for obsessive-compulsive symptoms. Fluoxetine, sertraline, and fluvoxamine all have evidence supporting their use in pediatric OCD. For children with PANDAS and PANS, initial doses should typically be lower than standard starting doses, with gradual titration as tolerated.

Antipsychotic medications, particularly those with dopamine-blocking properties like risperidone and aripiprazole, may help with severe tics, agitation, or aggression. However, their side effect profile — including weight gain, metabolic changes, and movement abnormalities, warrants careful consideration, particularly in a population that may already be predisposed to movement problems.

Medications for anxiety, attention, and sleep may be helpful for managing these common comorbid symptoms. Clonidine and guanfacine, alpha-2 agonists used for ADHD and tics, are often well tolerated and may help with anxiety, sleep, and attention in addition to their effects on tics. Melatonin is commonly used for sleep difficulties and is generally safe.

The integration of immunological and psychiatric approaches represents a change in thinking in treatment. Rather than viewing these as competing perspectives, clinicians increasingly recognize them as complementary. A child with PANDAS may benefit simultaneously from antibiotic prophylaxis, periodic IVIG infusions, ongoing cognitive behavioral therapy, a serotonin reuptake inhibitor, melatonin for sleep, and school accommodations. The combination addresses multiple aspects of the illness and likely produces better outcomes than any single intervention alone.

Treatment is typically ongoing and dynamic. As children mature and their immune systems change, the pattern of illness may shift. Flares become less frequent for many, and the intensity of immunomodulatory treatment may be able to decrease over time. For others, adolescence brings new challenges as hormonal changes affect immune function. Continued monitoring and adjustment of treatment is necessary throughout development.

THE ADULT DIMENSION: **Treating Psychoimmunological Disorders in Grown-Ups**

While PANDAS is by definition a pediatric condition, psychoimmunological disorders do not respect birthdays. Adults may experience new-onset autoimmune-mediated psychiatric illness, or they may be dealing with the long-term consequences of childhood-onset disease.

Adults who develop autoimmune encephalitis—anti-NMDA receptor encephalitis or related conditions—typically require aggressive immunomodulatory treatment and often hospitalization. The treatment approach is similar to that used in children: removing any triggering tumor if present, using immunotherapy (corticosteroids, IVIG, plasmapheresis, and sometimes rituximab or other immunosuppressive medications), and providing supportive care including management of psychiatric symptoms. Many patients recover substantially, though the process may take months to years and some experience lasting deficits.

For adults whose psychiatric illness has a suspected autoimmune component without meeting criteria for frank encephalitis, the approach is less well established. Some clinicians trial anti-inflammatory treatments in patients with treatment-resistant depression or psychosis who have elevated inflammatory markers or other suggestions of immune involvement. This remains an area of active research rather than established practice.

Adults with histories of childhood PANDAS or PANS may continue to benefit from the immunomodulatory approaches they used as children, or they may find that their illness has evolved into a more typical psychiatric condition that responds to standard treatments. The transition from pediatric to adult care is often challenging, as adult psychiatrists may be less familiar with psycho-immunological concepts than their pediatric colleagues.

In older adults, the intersection of immune function and brain health becomes particularly relevant to cognitive aging and dementia. Anti-inflammatory strategies, including both medications and lifestyle factors such as diet and exercise that affect inflammation, are being investigated for prevention and treatment of cognitive decline.

The field remains in early stages, but the recognition that immune function affects brain function across the lifespan opens new avenues for intervention.

THE FRONTIER AHEAD: **Where Psychoimmunology Meets the Future**

The discovery that immune processes can cause psychiatric symptoms has implications extending far beyond PANDAS and PANS. We are witnessing the early stages of a fundamental reconceptualization of mental illness—one that promises new diagnostic approaches, novel treatments, and perhaps even prevention strategies.

Precision diagnostics represent one frontier. As we identify more autoantibodies and inflammatory markers associated with psychiatric symptoms, we move toward the possibility of diagnostic tests that can identify patients whose illness has an immune component. Rather than treating all patients with depression identically, we might someday identify those whose depression is driven by inflammation and target that inflammation directly, while using different approaches for patients whose depression has other causes. Blood tests, cerebrospinal fluid analysis, and advanced brain imaging may all contribute to more precise diagnosis.

Novel therapeutics are already emerging from psychoimmunological research. Medications targeting specific inflammatory pathways, rather than broadly suppressing immune function, could provide the benefits of immunomodulation with fewer side effects. Biologics developed for other autoimmune conditions—medications targeting specific cytokines or immune cell types—are being investigated for psychiatric applications. The medication market of the future may include drugs designed specifically for immune-mediated psychiatric illness.

Microbiome-based approaches represent another avenue. The gut microbiome- the community of trillions of bacteria and other microorganisms living in our intestines—profoundly affects immune function and, through pathways still being elucidated, brain function as well. Manipulating the microbiome through diet, probiotics, or other interventions may offer new ways to modulate immune-brain interactions. Early research suggests that gut bacteria may influence autoimmune responses, though clinical applications remain largely theoretical.

Vaccine development might someday offer prevention of some psycho-immunological disorders. If certain infections trigger autoimmune brain disease, preventing those infections could prevent the psychiatric consequences. A vaccine against group A streptococcus has been a long-sought goal for decades, primarily to prevent rheumatic heart disease; if achieved, it might also reduce the incidence of PANDAS. Similar logic might apply to other infection-triggered psychiatric conditions.

Personalized medicine approaches will likely become increasingly important. Not everyone exposed to streptococcus develops PANDAS; genetic and other factors determine susceptibility. Identifying those at risk could enable targeted prevention or early intervention. Understanding why some individuals develop autoimmune brain disease while others do not may reveal fundamental insights into immune regulation that have broad applications.

Perhaps most profoundly, the psycho-immunological revolution is dissolving the artificial boundary between mind and body that has shaped Western medicine for centuries. The idea that psychiatric illness is fundamentally different from other medical illness—rooted in some immaterial realm of mind rather than in the biology of the brain, giving way to recognition that brain and body are inextricably connected, that immune cells and neurons communicate constantly, and that mental health cannot be separated from physical health.

This reconceptualization has implications for how we structure healthcare, how we train physicians, and how we as a society understand mental illness. The psychiatrist of the future may need to be as comfortable ordering autoantibody panels and interpreting inflammatory markers as they are conducting psychotherapy and prescribing antidepressants. The internist and neurologist may need to recognize psychiatric presentations of medical illness. The walls between specialties, always somewhat artificial, may need to become more permeable.

For patients and families, the psycho-immunological perspective offers something precious: a framework for understanding symptoms that were previously baffling or stigmatized, and a pathway to treatments that address root causes rather than merely suppressing symptoms. The child who changes overnight is not becoming "crazy" or acting out—something has gone wrong in her immune system, and with proper treatment, she can recover. This understanding does not diminish the reality of the suffering or the difficulty of the journey, but it does provide hope grounded in biological reality.

CONCLUSION: **The Body in the Mind**

We began this chapter with a child who changed overnight, her brain seemingly hijacked by forces beyond her control. We have traced the long history of observations linking infection and inflammation to mental symptoms, explored the mechanisms by which the immune system can turn against the brain, and examined how PANDAS, PANS, and related conditions are diagnosed and treated. We have seen how psycho-immunological processes operate across the lifespan, from childhood through old age, and glimpsed the future of a field that promises to transform our understanding of mental illness.

The central insight is simple but profound: the brain is part of the body. It is subject to the same inflammatory processes, the same immune attacks, the same infectious assaults that affect every other organ. When the immune system errs, the brain may suffer. When infection invades, the mind may fall ill. The apparent chasm between psychiatric and medical illness was always illusory; we are only now developing the tools and concepts to bridge it.

For families navigating PANDAS, PANS, or related conditions, this understanding offers a framework for making sense of bewildering symptoms and advocating for appropriate care. The journey is often difficult—finding knowledgeable providers, obtaining insurance coverage for treatments still considered experimental by some, managing the day-to-day challenges of caring for a child with episodic severe illness. But the path is clearer now than it was a generation ago, and it continues to become clearer as research advances.

For the broader field of psychiatry and for society as a whole, psychoimmunology represents a fundamental expansion of how we understand mental illness. Not all psychiatric illness has an immune component, but some do, and our treatments must evolve accordingly. The medications of the future may look very different from those of today. The diagnostic process may involve laboratory tests and biomarkers rather than relying solely on symptom checklists. The integration of mental health care with the rest of medicine may finally become reality rather than aspiration.

The child who changed overnight can change again—this time, for the better. Her immune system's misdirected attack on her brain can be calmed. Her obsessions and tics can fade. Her joy and confidence can return. The story that began in terror can end in recovery.

This is the promise of psychoimmunology: not merely a new way of understanding mental illness, but a new way of treating it, a new hope for those who suffer, and a new chapter in medicine's long effort to heal the whole person—body and mind together.

KEY POINTS for Patients and Families

PANDAS is a condition in which streptococcal infection triggers sudden-onset obsessive-compulsive disorder, tics, and related symptoms in children. PANS is a broader category that includes similar sudden-onset symptoms triggered by other infections or unknown causes.

The dramatic, overnight onset of symptoms is the hallmark of these conditions and distinguishes them from typical psychiatric disorders that develop gradually.

Diagnosis is clinical, based on the characteristic symptom pattern, temporal relationship to infection, and exclusion of other causes. No single test definitively confirms the diagnosis.

Common accompanying symptoms include severe anxiety, mood instability, cognitive problems, sleep disturbances, eating difficulties, and sensory sensitivities.

Treatment typically involves addressing any acute infection, using anti-inflammatory or immunomodulatory treatments to calm the immune response, and managing psychiatric symptoms with therapy and sometimes medication.

For severe cases, treatments like intravenous immunoglobulin (IVIG) or plasmapheresis may be recommended by specialists.

These conditions can persist through adolescence and adulthood, and similar autoimmune mechanisms may contribute to psychiatric illness at any age.

The recognition that immune processes can cause psychiatric symptoms is driving research into new diagnostics and treatments that may benefit many patients in the future.

QUESTIONS for Your Healthcare Provider

1. Could my child's sudden symptom onset suggest PANDAS or PANS?
2. Should we test for streptococcal infection or other infections?
3. What inflammatory or autoimmune testing might be helpful?
4. Would anti-inflammatory treatment be appropriate, and if so, what would you recommend?
5. Should we consider consultation with a specialist familiar with PANDAS and PANS?
6. What psychiatric treatments would you recommend for symptom management?
7. How will we monitor for infection triggers and prevent future flares?
8. What school accommodations should we request?
9. Are there clinical trials or research studies that might be appropriate?
10. How should we plan for transition to adult care if symptoms persist?

13

THE NEW PHARMACOLOGY OF THE MIND

FROM BLUNT INSTRUMENTS TO PRECISION TOOLS

A Revolution Quietly Unfolding

F or more than half a century, the treatment of mental illness has relied on a remarkably small set of pharmaceutical approaches. Medications that enhance serotonin signaling treat depression. Medications that block dopamine receptors treat psychosis. Medications that enhance GABA signaling treat anxiety. Stimulants that boost dopamine and norepinephrine treat attention deficit disorders. These drugs have helped millions of people, and their discovery ranks among the great achievements of twentieth-century medicine.

Yet anyone who has taken psychiatric medication or watched a loved one struggle to find the right treatment, knows the limitations of our current arsenal. The first antidepressant works well for only about one-third of patients; many must try multiple medications over months or years before finding one that helps. Side effects—weight gain, sexual dysfunction, emotional blunting, sedation—lead many patients to stop taking medications that are partially helping them. For some conditions, like the negative symptoms of schizophrenia or treatment-resistant depression, our existing medications offer only modest benefit at best. The gap between what psychiatric medications can do and what patients need them to do remains vast.

We stand now at the threshold of a new era. Advances in neuroscience, genetics, immunology, and pharmacology are converging to create possibilities that would have seemed fantastical just a generation ago. Psychedelic compounds once dismissed as dangerous drugs of abuse are demonstrating remarkable efficacy in clinical trials. Medications targeting entirely new brain systems are entering development. Genetic testing promises to guide treatment selection. Immunological approaches, as we explored in the previous chapter, are opening new therapeutic avenues. The field of psychopharmacology is being reinvented from the ground up.

This chapter explores the future of medication treatment for mental illness—the new drugs emerging from laboratories and clinical trials, the new understanding of brain function that is guiding their development, and the new approaches to treatment that may transform outcomes for patients who have not been well served by existing options. We will examine what is already here, what is coming soon, and what remains on the more distant horizon. Throughout, we will maintain appropriate humility about predictions in a field that has repeatedly surprised even its most knowledgeable practitioners.

The Limits of What We Have

To appreciate where psychopharmacology is heading, we must first understand honestly where it has been and where it stands today. The major classes of psychiatric medication were discovered largely by accident between the 1950s and 1980s. Chlorpromazine, the first antipsychotic, was initially developed as an antihistamine and anesthetic adjunct; its antipsychotic properties were noticed serendipitously. Imipramine, the first tricyclic antidepressant, was being tested as an antipsychotic when its mood-elevating effects became apparent. Lithium's antimanic properties were discovered when an Australian psychiatrist observed that guinea pigs became calm after receiving lithium injections.

These accidental discoveries launched a pharmaceutical revolution. For the first time, severe mental illnesses that had previously meant lifelong institutionalization could be treated. Patients with schizophrenia could leave hospitals and live in the community. Patients with depression could find relief from suffering that had seemed unending. The medications were imperfect—side effects were often severe, and not everyone responded—but they represented an enormous advance over what had come before.

The decades that followed brought refinements rather than fundamental breakthroughs. The selective serotonin reuptake inhibitors, or SSRIs, introduced in the late 1980s, offered a more tolerable side effect profile than older antidepressants but were not more effective. Second-generation antipsychotics reduced some neurological side effects but introduced metabolic problems. The basic mechanisms—enhancing monoamine neurotransmission for depression, blocking dopamine for psychosis—remained unchanged. We got better at deploying the same tools, but we did not develop fundamentally new ones.

This long drought of innovation had multiple causes. The brain proved far more complex than early models suggested, and the simple "chemical imbalance" theories that guided early drug development turned out to be vast oversimplifications. Drug development became increasingly expensive and risky, with many promising compounds failing in late-stage clinical trials. Pharmaceutical companies, burned by costly failures, retreated from neuroscience research, leaving the field underfunded relative to other areas of medicine.

The consequences for patients have been significant. Consider depression, the most common condition treated with psychiatric medication. Standard antidepressants work by increasing the availability of serotonin, norepinephrine, or both in the synapses between neurons. Yet these changes in neurotransmitter levels occur within hours of taking the medication, while clinical improvement typically takes weeks. This temporal mismatch suggests that the immediate neurochemical effects are not directly responsible for improvement—something downstream, some slower adaptation of neural circuits, must be doing the actual therapeutic work. We prescribe these medications based on a theory we know to be incomplete.

Moreover, standard antidepressants simply do not work for everyone. The landmark STAR*D trial, which followed patients through multiple sequential medication trials, found that about one-third of patients achieved remission with their first antidepressant, another quarter or so with a second trial, and progressively fewer with subsequent trials. After four sequential treatment attempts, about one-third of patients still had not achieved remission. These treatment-resistant patients—and there are millions of them—have been waiting for something better.

For other conditions, the limitations are equally stark. The positive symptoms of schizophrenia—hallucinations and delusions—often respond to antipsychotic medications, but the negative symptoms—social withdrawal, emotional flatness, lack of motivation—and the cognitive symptoms—difficulty with memory, attention, and executive function—respond poorly if at all. Since negative and cognitive symptoms are often more disabling than positive symptoms for long-term functioning, this represents a major gap in treatment.

Anxiety disorders often improve with SSRIs, but improvement may be partial and accompanied by troubling side effects. Many patients prefer benzodiazepines, which work quickly and reliably, but these carry risks of dependence and cognitive impairment that limit their long-term use. We lack medications that provide rapid, reliable anxiety relief without these downsides.

Bipolar disorder, post-traumatic stress disorder, obsessive-compulsive disorder, eating disorders—for each, our current medications offer meaningful help to some patients while leaving others inadequately treated. The field has been candid about these limitations; the question is what to do about them.

KETAMINE and the Glutamate Revolution

The first genuinely new mechanism for treating depression in decades came from an unexpected source: ketamine, a decade-old anesthetic with a reputation as a club drug. In the late 1990s and early 2000s, researchers began investigating whether ketamine, which works on the brain's glutamate system rather than the serotonin system, might have antidepressant effects. What they found was remarkable.

Ketamine produced antidepressant effects within hours—not the weeks required for traditional antidepressants. For patients who had not responded to multiple other medications, ketamine offered rapid relief. The effect was not subtle; patients who had been severely depressed and sometimes suicidal, experienced significant improvement after a single infusion. Studies replicated these findings again and again. Something genuinely new was happening.

The glutamate system, which ketamine affects, is the brain's primary excitatory neurotransmitter system. Glutamate signaling is fundamental to learning, memory, and the strengthening and weakening of synaptic connections that underlies neural plasticity. Ketamine blocks one type of glutamate receptor, the NMDA receptor, but its antidepressant effects likely involve complex downstream consequences including enhanced plasticity and the growth of new synaptic connections.

The rapidity of ketamine's effects suggested that depression might not require weeks of gradual neurochemical rebalancing to improve. Instead, something like a reset of neural circuit function might be possible—a rapid shift from a depressed state to a healthier one. This conceptual shift opened new ways of thinking about treatment.

Ketamine itself, however, has significant limitations. It must be administered intravenously or by injection for reliable absorption, making treatment inconvenient and expensive. Its effects are dissociative patients may feel detached from reality, experience perceptual distortions, or have out-of-body experiences during treatment. While generally safe under medical supervision, ketamine has abuse potential and can cause problems with repeated heavy use. Its antidepressant effects, while rapid, are also often temporary, requiring repeated treatments to maintain improvement.

These limitations spurred development of related compounds. Esketamine, a variant of ketamine administered as a nasal spray, received FDA approval in 2019 for treatment-resistant depression and later for depression with suicidal ideation. The nasal spray formulation improved convenience, though treatment still requires administration in a healthcare setting with monitoring. Esketamine represented the first approval of a fundamentally new mechanism for depression in decades—a proof of concept that the glutamate system could be therapeutically targeted.

Research continues into other glutamate-targeting compounds that might offer ketamine's benefits with fewer drawbacks. Some compounds target the same NMDA receptors through different mechanisms. Others target different glutamate receptors entirely. The goal is to capture the rapid antidepressant effect and enhanced neural plasticity while minimizing dissociation, abuse potential, and the need for clinical supervision.

Beyond depression, glutamate-targeting medications are being investigated for other conditions. Obsessive-compulsive disorder, which often responds incompletely to serotonin-based treatments, has shown promising responses to glutamate-modulating drugs in some studies. Anxiety disorders, PTSD, and even schizophrenia are being examined through glutamate lens.

The ketamine story illustrates several themes that recur throughout the new psychopharmacology. A compound with an entirely different mechanism from existing treatments proved effective where those treatments had failed. Rapid effects challenged assumptions that improvement required slow neuroadaptation. And the path from initial discovery to approved medication, while eventually successful, required overcoming skepticism rooted in the compound's unconventional history and effects.

Psychedelics: From Counterculture to Clinic

Perhaps no development in psychiatry has attracted more public attention than the renaissance of psychedelic-assisted therapy. Compounds like psilocybin (the active ingredient in "magic mushrooms"), MDMA (the empathogen often called ecstasy or molly), and LSD, banned for decades and associated in the public mind with the excesses of the 1960s counterculture, are now subjects of rigorous clinical trials at major academic medical centers. The results have been remarkable enough to prompt FDA designation as break-through therapies and to suggest that psychedelic-assisted treatment may become available for certain conditions within the next few years.

The history of psychedelic research has been tumultuous. In the 1950s and 1960s, thousands of patients received LSD and other psychedelics in clinical settings, with promising results reported for alcoholism, depression, and end-of-life anxiety. However, the cultural and political upheaval associated with recreational psychedelic use led to their classification as Schedule I controlled substances, effectively halting research. For decades, these compounds were scientifically radioactive—too associated with counterculture to be taken seriously.

The renaissance began quietly in the 1990s and 2000s, as a small group of researchers obtained permission to conduct carefully controlled studies. What they found confirmed what earlier researchers had suggested: in the right setting, with appropriate preparation and support, psychedelic experiences could produce profound and lasting therapeutic benefits.

Psilocybin has been studied most extensively for depression and for existential distress in patients facing terminal illness. Multiple trials have found that one or two psilocybin sessions, combined with psychological support before, during, and after the experience, produce large and sustained improvements in depression symptoms. In studies of patients with life-threatening cancer diagnoses, psilocybin reduced anxiety and depression related to mortality and improved quality of life, with effects lasting months after a single session. The magnitude of improvement in these studies has been striking—larger than typically seen with conventional antidepressants.

MDMA has been studied primarily for post-traumatic stress

disorder, a condition notoriously difficult to treat. MDMA increases feelings of emotional closeness and reduces fear responses, potentially creating a window in which traumatic memories can be processed without overwhelming distress. Phase 3 trials found that MDMA-assisted therapy produced substantially better outcomes than therapy alone, with a majority of participants no longer meeting criteria for PTSD after treatment. These results led the FDA to consider approval, though the process has involved complexities reflecting the novel nature of this treatment approach.

What makes psychedelic-assisted therapy distinctive is that the drug is not taken daily like conventional medication. Instead, one or a few carefully supervised sessions are embedded within a broader therapeutic process. Preparation sessions establish trust and set intentions. The medication session itself lasts several hours, with therapists present to provide support. Integration sessions afterward help patients make sense of their experiences and translate insights into lasting change. The drug facilitates a process, but the process itself—the preparation, presence of trained therapists, the integration—is essential to outcomes.

The experiences produced by psychedelics are difficult to describe but often involve a sense of profound meaningfulness, dissolution of ordinary ego boundaries, feelings of connection to something larger than oneself, and emotionally intense revisiting of significant memories or concerns. These experiences appear to facilitate psychological flexibility, allowing patients to see their problems from new perspectives and make changes they had been unable to make before.

The neuroscience of psychedelic effects is an active research area. Psilocybin and LSD work primarily through serotonin 2A receptors, but their effects on brain network connectivity may be more relevant to their therapeutic impact. Neuroimaging studies show that psychedelics temporarily disrupt the normal hierarchical organization of brain activity, potentially allowing new patterns of connectivity to emerge. This may relate to the sense of expanded possibilities and the ability to break out of rigid thought patterns that characterize the therapeutic response.

Challenges remain in translating psychedelic-assisted therapy from research settings to clinical practice. The treatment model requires extensive therapist time and training, specialized facilities, and careful patient selection and monitoring. Scaling these requirements to meet potential demand presents logistical challenges. There are also unresolved questions about which patients are most likely to benefit, how to handle adverse psychological reactions during sessions, and how to integrate this approach within existing healthcare systems.

Regulatory pathways are evolving to accommodate these novel treatments. MDMA-assisted therapy has faced regulatory scrutiny not only for the drug itself but for the therapy protocol and the potential for therapist misconduct in emotionally intense treatment settings. Psilocybin is being considered for approval in various jurisdictions, with Oregon and Colorado having already created frameworks for supervised psilocybin services. The FDA and other regulators are navigating unprecedented questions about how to evaluate treatments where set and setting matter as much as the compound itself.

Despite these challenges, the psychedelic renaissance represents a fundamental shift in psychiatric treatment. For patients with treatment-resistant depression, PTSD, end-of-life distress, and potentially other conditions, these approaches offer possibilities that did not exist a decade ago. The coming years will determine how widely accessible these treatments become and how they are integrated with other psychiatric care.

. . .

TARGETING the Brain's Inflammation

As we explored in the previous chapter, immune and inflammatory processes contribute to psychiatric symptoms in some patients. This understanding is now driving medication development aimed specifically at the immune-brain interface.

The evidence that inflammation contributes to at least some depression has become substantial. Subsets of depressed patients have elevated inflammatory markers in their blood. Patients given inflammatory cytokines for medical treatment often develop depressive symptoms. Anti-inflammatory treatments have shown antidepressant effects in some trials, particularly in patients with elevated baseline inflammation. These observations suggest that for some patients, depression may be as much an inflammatory condition as a neurochemical one.

Medications that specifically target inflammatory pathways are now being investigated for depression and other psychiatric conditions. These include drugs originally developed for rheumatoid arthritis, inflammatory bowel disease, or psoriasis—conditions characterized by excessive inflammation. Early trials have shown mixed but intriguing results, with benefit appearing most clearly in patients who had elevated inflammation before treatment. This makes biological sense: if inflammation is contributing to symptoms, reducing inflammation should help; if it is not, anti-inflammatory treatment would not be expected to produce psychiatric improvement.

The challenge is identifying which patients have inflammation-driven psychiatric illness. Simple blood tests for inflammatory markers can help, but current markers are neither sensitive nor specific enough for reliable patient selection. Research is ongoing to develop better biomarkers that can identify patients likely to benefit from anti-inflammatory approaches.

Beyond depression, inflammatory mechanisms are being investigated in schizophrenia, bipolar disorder, obsessive-compulsive disorder, and autism spectrum disorder. The specific inflammatory pathways involved may differ across conditions, suggesting that different anti-inflammatory strategies may be needed for different disorders.

Microglial modulation represents a more targeted approach. Microglia are the brain's resident immune cells, responsible for surveillance, debris clearance, and inflammatory responses within the central nervous system. When activated excessively, microglia may contribute to neuronal damage and psychiatric symptoms. Medications that reduce excessive microglial activation while preserving their necessary functions could potentially treat neuroinflammatory psychiatric illness with fewer systemic effects than drugs targeting inflammation throughout the body.

The gut-brain axis offers another avenue for immune modulation. The gut microbiome—the community of bacteria, fungi, and other microorganisms living in the intestinal tract—profoundly influences immune function and, through various pathways, brain function. Alterations in the gut microbiome have been associated with depression, anxiety, and other psychiatric conditions. Probiotics, prebiotics, dietary changes, and even fecal microbiota transplantation are being investigated as means to shift the gut microbiome toward healthier configurations that might reduce inflammation and improve mental health. While this field remains in early stages, with more questions than answers, the potential for safe, accessible microbiome-based interventions is exciting.

These inflammatory and immune approaches are not meant to replace existing treatments but to complement them. A patient whose depression has an inflammatory component might benefit from an anti-inflammatory medication added to their antidepressant —addressing two different aspects of their illness simultaneously. The goal is precision rather than replacement, matching treatments to the specific mechanisms operating in each individual patient.

Neuroplasticity: **Medications That Help the Brain Change**

One of the most exciting frontiers in psychopharmacology involves medications that enhance the brain's capacity to change—its neuroplasticity. Rather than directly correcting a chemical imbalance or blocking a disease process, these medications make the brain more responsive to experience, more capable of learning new patterns and unlearning maladaptive ones. When combined with psychotherapy or other behavioral interventions, they may accelerate and deepen therapeutic change.

The concept has precedent in the ketamine story. Part of ketamine's rapid antidepressant effect appears to involve enhanced synaptic plasticity-the growth of new connections between neurons and the strengthening of beneficial circuit patterns. The dissociative experience may matter less than this biological priming of the brain for change.

Psychedelics likely work through similar mechanisms. The profound experiences they produce occur against a background of enhanced neural plasticity, allowing new insights to become durably encoded. This may explain why the effects of a single psychedelic session can persist for months—the brain was changed in ways that outlast the acute drug effects.

Research is now exploring compounds that enhance plasticity without producing the dramatic altered states of ketamine or psychedelics. Brain-derived neurotrophic factor, or BDNF, is a protein that promotes neuron survival, growth, and plasticity. Many effective treatments for depression—including antidepressants, exercise, and electroconvulsive therapy—increase BDNF levels. Drugs that directly enhance BDNF signaling or related pathways could potentially accelerate therapeutic change.

Other targets include receptors and signaling molecules involved in learning and memory. AMPA receptors, a type of glutamate receptor, play a central role in synaptic strengthening. Positive allosteric modulators of AMPA receptors—drugs that enhance the receptors' function without directly activating them—are being developed as potential cognitive enhancers and antidepressants. Early results have been mixed, but the concept remains promising.

The critical insight driving this research is that psychiatric illness often involves learned patterns of thought, emotion, and behavior that have become entrenched. Fear responses in PTSD, ruminative thought patterns in depression, compulsive behaviors in OCD—all represent neural circuits that have become rigid and maladaptive. Medications that enhance plasticity could potentially help patients break out of these patterns, especially when combined with therapy that guides the learning of healthier alternatives.

This suggests a model of treatment very different from current practice. Rather than taking a medication daily for maintenance of effect, patients might take a plasticity-enhancing medication at specific times—perhaps during therapy sessions or during intensive treatment programs—to maximize the durability of therapeutic gains. The medication becomes an adjunct to experiential learning rather than a primary treatment.

Early studies of this approach are beginning to appear. D-cycloserine, an old antibiotic that also affects glutamate receptors, has been studied as an adjunct to exposure therapy for anxiety disorders. When taken before exposure sessions, it appears to enhance fear extinction learning, helping patients more thoroughly unlearn their fear responses. Results have been inconsistent across studies, suggesting that the approach may work for some patients or require specific conditions to be effective, but the principle has been demonstrated.

Researchers are also exploring whether medications can enhance the effects of behavioral interventions for conditions beyond anxiety. Could this plasticity-enhancing medication make cognitive remediation more effective for patients with schizophrenia? Could it help patients with addiction more thoroughly learn to resist triggers? Could it improve outcomes from couples therapy or parent training? These questions await research, but they illustrate the broad potential of the neuroplasticity approach.

Precision Psychiatry: The Right Drug for the Right Patient

One of the most frustrating aspects of current psychiatric treatment is the trial-and-error process of finding the right medication. Patients try one drug, wait weeks to see if it works, experience side effects, try another, wait again—a process that can stretch over months or years while symptoms persist. What if we could predict from the start which medication would work best for each individual patient?

This is the promise of precision psychiatry, also called personalized or stratified medicine. Rather than treating all patients with a given diagnosis identically, precision psychiatry aims to match treatments to the biological characteristics of individual patients. Several approaches are being developed toward this goal.

Pharmacogenomics uses genetic testing to predict how patients will respond to specific medications. Genetic variations affect the enzymes that metabolize drugs, the receptors that drugs target, and other aspects of drug response. Some patients are "rapid metaboliz-ers" who break down certain drugs so quickly that standard doses are ineffective; others are "poor metabolizers" for whom standard doses produce excessive blood levels and side effects. Knowing a patient's genetic profile can help select medications and doses more likely to be effective and well tolerated.

The FDA has approved pharmacogenomic labels for many psychiatric medications, indicating genetic factors that may affect response. Commercial tests are available that provide guidance on medication selection based on genetic profiles. However, the clinical utility of these tests remains debated. While they clearly identify some patients at risk for adverse effects or inadequate response, the improvement in overall outcomes from routine pharmacogenomic testing has been modest in clinical trials conducted to date. The tests may be most useful for specific clinical situations—patients who have failed multiple trials, patients who have experienced unusual side effects, patients with complex polypharmacy—rather than for all patients starting treatment.

Beyond pharmacogenomics, researchers are developing biomarkers that might predict treatment response based on other biological characteristics. Brain imaging studies have identified patterns of neural activity that predict response to medication versus psychotherapy, or to one class of medication versus another. Inflam-matory markers might identify patients who are likely to respond to anti-inflammatory approaches. Electroencephalography, or EEG, patterns have shown some ability to predict antidepressant response. Combining multiple biomarkers—genetic, imaging, blood-based, and clinical—into predictive algorithms is an active area of research.

Machine learning and artificial intelligence are being applied to psychiatric prediction problems. By analyzing large datasets of patient characteristics and outcomes, algorithms can identify patterns too complex for human clinicians to detect. Some of these algorithms have shown impressive accuracy in predicting treatment response in research settings. Whether they will prove useful in real-world clinical practice remains to be demonstrated as they are tested more widely.

The ultimate vision of precision psychiatry is a future in which treatment selection is guided by comprehensive biological assessment. A patient presenting with depression would undergo genetic testing, perhaps blood tests for inflammatory and other markers, possibly brief brain imaging or EEG, and clinical assessment. An algorithm would integrate this data with information about available treatments and their likely effects in similar patients, producing a ranked list of treatment recommendations. The clinician would discuss these recommendations with the patient, incorporate patient preferences and practical considerations, and select a treatment with much higher probability of success than current trial-and-error approaches.

We are not yet near this turn in the future, but we are moving toward it. Each research study that identifies predictors of treatment response, each new biomarker validated, each algorithm refined, brings us closer. Within the next decade, precision psychiatry is likely to become increasingly practical for at least some clinical decisions, even if the comprehensive vision remains further away.

DIGITAL THERAPEUTICS and Drug-Device Combinations

The boundary between medication and other forms of treatment is blurring. Digital therapeutic software applications that deliver therapeutic interventions—are beginning to be prescribed alongside or instead of medications. Some are being developed in combination with drugs to produce synergistic effects.

Several digital therapeutics have received FDA authorization for psychiatric conditions. Apps delivering cognitive behavioral therapy for insomnia, attention training for ADHD, and therapeutic content for substance use disorders have passed regulatory review and are being prescribed by physicians. These represent a new category of treatment—software as medicine—with its own evidence requirements, regulatory pathways, and clinical considerations.

The combination of medications and digital therapeutics may prove particularly powerful. A medication that enhances neuroplasticity, for instance, could be combined with a digital program that delivers therapeutic exercises, potentially producing better outcomes than either used alone. Medication makes the brain more changeable; the digital program guides the direction of that change. This combination approach is being studied for anxiety, depression, and other conditions.

Closed-loop systems that monitor patients and adjust treatment in real time represent a more futuristic application. Imagine a smartwatch that monitors physiological indicators of mood or anxiety and detects warning signs, prompts therapeutic exercises, or alerts the patient's care team. More aggressively, imagine a system that could adjust medication delivery based on continuous monitoring—increasing an anti-anxiety medication during periods of detected high stress, for instance, or alerting to early mood episode onset. Such systems are technically feasible and are being developed, though clinical validation and regulatory approval remain ahead.

Neuromodulation devices that directly stimulate brain activity are another frontier. Transcranial magnetic stimulation, or TMS, uses magnetic fields to stimulate specific brain regions and is already approved for treatment-resistant depression. Newer devices offer more targeted stimulation, home-based treatment, or combination with other interventions. Deep brain stimulation, which involves surgically implanted electrodes, is being studied for severe treatment-resistant depression and OCD. Less invasive approaches like transcranial direct current stimulation are being explored for various conditions.

These device-based approaches can be combined with medications in various ways. A patient might receive TMS to address treatment-resistant depression while also taking medication and engaging in psychotherapy. The different modalities may work through complementary mechanisms, producing benefits unavailable from any single approach.

The integration of digital tools, devices, and medications into comprehensive treatment plans represents a significant departure from the traditional model of picking a single drug and adjusting the dose. Treatment increasingly resembles a customized combination of interventions selected to address the specific needs of each patient—a far cry from the one-size-fits-all approach of earlier eras.

New Targets, New Molecules

Basic neuroscience research continues to identify potential targets for psychiatric medication development. While not all will pan out, the pipeline of candidates is more robust than it was a decade ago, and several promising directions merit attention.

The endocannabinoid system, which modulates stress responses, mood, and many other functions, is one target of active interest. The brain produces its own cannabis-like molecules that regulate neural signaling. Medications that enhance endocannabinoid signaling, without producing the intoxication associated with cannabis itself, could potentially treat anxiety, PTSD, and possibly depression. Some compounds in development show promise in early trials, though the path to approved medications remains uncertain.

Orexin receptors, which regulate sleep and arousal, are another target. Orexin-blocking medications are already approved for insomnia. Research is exploring whether modulation of this system might help with other conditions, including depression, anxiety, and addiction.

Kappa opioid receptors have been linked to dysphoria and depression. Unlike the mu opioid receptors targeted by drugs like morphine and heroin, kappa receptors produce unpleasant rather than euphoric effects when activated. Blocking these receptors might relieve depression without the addiction risk associated with traditional opioids. Several kappa antagonists are in development.

The psychedelic renaissance has renewed interest in serotonin 2A receptors, through which psilocybin and LSD produce their effects. Researchers are exploring whether compounds that activate these receptors with shorter duration of action, or that produce the beneficial effects without the full psychedelic experience, might offer therapeutic benefits with greater practicality.

Neurosteroids-steroid compounds produced in the brain that modulate neural activity—represent yet another avenue. Brexanolone, a neurosteroid that enhances GABA signaling, was approved in 2019 for postpartum depression, representing the first medication specifically developed and approved for this condition. Oral neurosteroid medications with broader applications are in development.

This sampling of targets barely scratches the surface of ongoing research. The brain contains hundreds of receptor types, thousands of signaling molecules, and networks of almost unfathomable complexity. As our understanding of this complexity deepens, new opportunities for intervention emerge.

. . .

THE INTEGRATION of **Psychopharmacology and Psychotherapy**

Throughout the history of modern psychiatry, a tension has existed between medication-focused and therapy-focused approaches. Some practitioners have emphasized biological intervention; others have insisted on the primacy of psychological treatment. Patients have often been caught between these camps, receiving one approach when they might benefit from both, or experiencing conflict between providers who advocate different strategies.

The new psychopharmacology dissolves this tension. The most promising emerging treatments are inherently integrative, requiring both pharmacological and psychological elements. Psychedelic-assisted therapy is meaningless without the therapy. Plasticity-enhancing medications work by facilitating learning that must be guided by experience. Even traditional medications increasingly appear to work partly by enabling the brain changes that therapy produces.

This integration has practical implications. The psychiatrist who prescribes medication and the therapist who provides psychological treatment must communicate and coordinate. Treatment planning must consider how different modalities might complement each other. Patients must understand that medication and therapy are partners, not alternatives.

Training implications follow. Psychiatrists need enough understanding of psychotherapy to collaborate effectively with therapists and to recognize when psychological treatment is essential. Psychologists and other therapists need enough understanding of medication mechanisms to participate meaningfully in integrated treatment planning. Interdisciplinary collaboration, long advocated but often poorly implemented, becomes truly necessary.

New treatment settings may be required. Psychedelic-assisted therapy cannot be delivered in a traditional fifteen-minute medication management appointment or a fifty-minute therapy session. It requires specialized facilities, extended time, and integrated medical and psychological supervision. Ketamine treatment similarly requires infrastructure that many practices lack. As novel treatments become available, the healthcare system must adapt to deliver them.

Access, Equity, and the Future of Psychiatric Treatment

Advances in psychiatric treatment are meaningless if patients cannot access them. The history of psychiatric care includes too many instances of promising treatments being available only to the privileged—those with excellent insurance, proximity to academic medical centers, or the resources to pay out of pocket.

The new psychopharmacology raises particular access concerns. Treatments like ketamine infusions and psychedelic-assisted therapy are expensive, typically costing thousands of dollars per session. They require specialized facilities and highly trained providers. Insurance coverage is inconsistent. For now, these treatments are available primarily to the wealthy.

Genetic testing and biomarker-based treatment selection could either reduce or exacerbate disparities. If precision psychiatry improves outcomes for all patients regardless of background, and if the tests are covered by insurance and available in community settings, it could reduce the current inequities in treatment success rates. But if precision approaches are available only to those who can afford expensive testing and specialty consultation, they could widen the gap between the psychiatric have and have-nots.

Digital therapeutics and telemedicine offer potential for democratizing access. A therapy app can reach patients in rural areas with no local therapist. An algorithm for treatment selection can guide clinicians without specialized training. These technologies could extend the benefits of advances to populations currently under-served. But they also require internet access, smartphone ownership, and digital literacy that not all patients have.

As new treatments emerge, deliberate attention to access and equity is essential. This includes research to develop effective lower-cost alternatives to expensive treatments, advocacy for insurance coverage, training programs that extend expertise beyond academic centers, and public health infrastructure that ensures all patients can benefit from advances regardless of their socioeconomic status.

Risks, Regulation, and the Responsible Path Forward

New treatments bring new risks. The history of medicine is littered with interventions that initially seemed promising but proved harmful—or that were beneficial for some patients but caused damage when used too broadly or carelessly.

Psychedelics illustrate complexity. While clinical trials show many remarkable benefits for carefully selected patients receiving treatment from well-trained therapists in controlled settings, these conditions are difficult to replicate in real-world practice. Patients with psychotic disorders or severe personality disorders may be harmed rather than helped. Poorly trained providers may fail to manage adverse reactions. The therapy component, essential to positive outcomes, may be diluted as treatment scales up. Ensuring that psychedelic-assisted therapy remains safe and effective as it moves from research to widespread practice is a major challenge.

The regulatory system is adapting to novel treatment approaches, but adaptation takes time and sometimes produces missteps. Regulators must balance the urgency of patients who need better options against the need for adequate evidence of safety and efficacy. They must develop frameworks for treatments that do not fit existing categories—drugs that work only in combination with therapy, digital therapeutics, closed-loop devices. Getting this balance right is crucial for ensuring that innovation benefits patients without exposing them to undue harm.

Individual practitioners bear responsibility for using new treatments appropriately. The temptation to offer the latest breakthrough can outrun evidence. Practitioners must honestly assess their own competence to deliver complex treatments and refer when they lack adequate training. They must resist pressure to expand indications beyond what evidence supports. First, doing no harm remains the essential principle.

Patients, too, have a role in navigating the new landscape. The promise of breakthrough treatments attracts hype, misinformation, and exploitation. Patients should seek treatment from qualified providers operating within evidence-based frameworks, ask questions about risks and alternatives, and maintain appropriate skepticism about claims that sound too good to be true.

Toward an Integrated Vision of Brain Health

The future of psychiatric treatment lies not only in new medications but in a transformed understanding of brain health as part of overall health—and of mental healthcare as part of healthcare generally. The artificial separation of mental and physical illness, of psychiatry from the rest of medicine, has been harmful to patients and limiting to science. That separation is finally breaking down.

As we have seen throughout this chapter and the one before, the brain is an organ affected by inflammation, infection, metabolism, hormones, and every other system of the body. Psychiatric symptoms can arise from immune attack, nutritional deficiency, hormonal imbalance, or genetic vulnerability—or, more commonly, from complex interactions among multiple factors. Treating psychiatric illness effectively requires understanding and addressing this full range of contributing causes.

The psychiatrist of the future will be as comfortable ordering autoantibody panels, reviewing brain imaging, and interpreting genetic tests as prescribing medications and coordinating therapy. The internist and primary care physician will recognize psychiatric symptoms as signals of potentially treatable underlying conditions, not merely problems to be referred away. Patients will understand that their mental health is not separate from their physical health, and that caring for their brains means caring for their bodies and minds together.

Lifestyle factors—sleep, exercise, diet, stress management, social connection—will be recognized not as supplements to treatment but as foundations of brain health. The evidence that these factors affect mood, cognition, and resilience is overwhelming and growing. Future treatment plans will integrate lifestyle intervention as systematically as medication.

Prevention will receive greater emphasis. Identifying individuals at risk for psychiatric illness and intervening before symptoms fully emerge may be possible as biomarkers and prediction algorithms improve. Early intervention in psychosis, for instance, has already been shown to improve long-term outcomes; similar approaches for mood disorders, anxiety, and other conditions may follow.

The vision, ultimately, is of healthcare that supports human flourishing across the lifespan—that helps people not merely survive but thrive, not merely avoid illness but cultivate wellbeing. Psychiatric treatment, in this vision, is not a separate domain concerned with a stigmatized category of illness but an integral part of caring for whole persons in all their complexity.

· · ·

CONCLUSION: **The Next Fifty Years**

Fifty years ago, we had a handful of psychiatric medications discovered largely by accident, working through mechanisms we barely understood, helpful for some patients and inadequate for many others. Today, we have the beginnings of a new pharmacology —new mechanisms like ketamine and psychedelics, new understanding of immune-brain interactions, new approaches to enhancing plasticity and personalizing treatment. The contrast is striking. Progress, though incomplete, is real.

Fifty years from now, what will psychiatric treatment look like? Predictions are hazardous, but some directions seem plausible.

We will likely have many more treatment options, targeting a much wider range of brain mechanisms. The monoamine-focused treatments that have dominated for decades will be supplemented by drugs affecting glutamate, neurosteroids, cannabinoids, inflammation, and systems not yet discovered.

We will likely match treatments to individual patients based on biological profiles, dramatically reducing the current trial-and-error process. Genetic testing, brain imaging, blood biomarkers, and clinical algorithms will guide treatment selection from the start.

We will likely integrate medication with psychotherapy in new ways, using plasticity-enhancing drugs to accelerate and deepen the learning that therapy produces. The opposition between biological and psychological approaches will seem as quaint as phrenology.

We will likely understand that many psychiatric conditions have subtypes with different underlying mechanisms, and we will treat these subtypes differently. "Depression" may prove to be as heterogeneous as "fever"—not a single disease but a common symptom of many different processes requiring different treatments.

We will likely have treatments that do more than reduce symptoms—that actively promote wellbeing, enhance resilience, and support human flourishing. Prevention will complement treatment.

None of this is guaranteed. Translating research into practice takes time, money, and sustained effort. Regulatory hurdles must be navigated. Access must be ensured. Mistakes will be made and lessons painfully learned. The history of medicine teaches humility about predictions.

But the direction is clear. The blunt instruments of twentieth-century psychopharmacology are giving way to the precision tools of twenty-first-century neuroscience. The artificial boundary between mental and physical illness is dissolving. The integration of biological, psychological, and social approaches to brain health is becoming reality.

For patients who have struggled with mental illness, for families who have watched loved ones suffer, for clinicians who have worked within the limitations of inadequate tools, this transformation offers hope. Not false hope—the journey remains difficult, and not all problems will be solved. But genuine hope, grounded in scientific progress and clinical evidence, that better treatments are coming. Some are already here. More are on the way.

The mind is part of the body. The brain is an organ. Mental illness is illness. And the future of treating it is brighter than it has ever been.

Key Points for Patients and Families

Current psychiatric medications help many people but have significant limitations, including delayed onset of effect, partial response for many patients, and troublesome side effects. New treatments are addressing these limitations.

Ketamine and related medications represent the first new mechanism for treating depression in decades, offering rapid-acting relief for some patients with treatment-resistant depression.

Psychedelic-assisted therapy, using compounds like psilocybin and MDMA combined with psychological support, has shown remarkable results in clinical trials for depression, PTSD, and end-of-life distress.

Immune and inflammatory processes contribute to psychiatric symptoms in some patients, opening new treatment avenues using anti-inflammatory and immunomodulatory approaches.

Medications that enhance neuroplasticity—the brain's capacity to change—may work by making the brain more responsive to therapy and positive experiences.

Precision psychiatry aims to match treatments to individual patients based on genetic and biological profiles, reducing the current trial-and-error approach to finding effective medication.

Digital therapeutics and device-based treatments are being combined with medications to produce enhanced effects.

Integration of medication with psychotherapy is increasingly recognized as optimal for many conditions, with each approach enhancing the other.

Access to new treatments remains a significant concern, with many advanced approaches currently available primarily to those with excellent insurance or financial resources.

QUESTIONS for Your Healthcare Provider

1. Am I a candidate for any of the newer treatment approaches, like ketamine or psychedelic-assisted therapy?

2. Would pharmacogenomic testing help guide me selection of medication?

3. Should we consider whether inflammation or immune factors might be contributing to my symptoms?

4. How might medication and therapy work together in my treatment plan?

5. Are there clinical trials for new treatments that I might be eligible for?

6. What lifestyle factors might support my brain health alongside medication?

7. How do we decide when to adjust my medication versus when to wait for fuller effect?

8. Are there digital therapeutics or apps that might complement my treatment?

9. What are the realistic expectations for improvement with available treatments?

10. How will we know if my current treatment is working well enough or if we should consider alternatives?

～

14

PSYCHOTHERAPY IN
THE MODERN ERA
ANCIENT WISDOM, NEW SCIENCE

The Talking Cure Reimagined

L ong before the first psychiatric medication was synthesized, humans discovered that conversation could heal. The confession to a priest, the counsel of an elder, the catharsis of sharing one's burdens with a trusted friend—these practices emerged across cultures and centuries because they worked. Something about putting suffering into words, about being heard and understood by another person, about gaining new perspective on one's troubles, produces relief that no physical remedy can match.

Modern psychotherapy represents the formalization and refinement of this ancient insight. Over the past century, clinicians and researchers have developed structured approaches to therapeutic conversation, tested them rigorously, and identified the elements that make them effective. What began as intuition has become science— though, as we shall see, the human elements that made informal helping relationships work remain central to even the most evidence-based modern treatments.

This chapter explores psychotherapy as it exists today and as it is evolving. We will examine the major approaches that research has validated, the common elements that make diverse therapies effective, the new technologies that are extending therapy's reach, and the integration of psychological treatment with the biological approaches covered in previous chapters. For patients considering therapy, family members trying to understand it, and anyone curious about how structured conversation produces lasting change, this chapter offers a map of the therapeutic landscape.

What Therapy Is—And What It Is Not

Misconceptions about psychotherapy abound. Some imagine therapy as an endless excavation of childhood memories, conducted on a leather couch while a bearded analyst takes notes. Others picture it as simply talking to a sympathetic listener who offers generic encouragement. Still others assume therapy is for people with severe mental illness, not ordinary people facing ordinary problems.

None of these images capture the reality of modern psychotherapy. Today's evidence-based treatments are typically focused, structured, and time-limited. They target specific problems using specific techniques. They are active—therapists teach skills, assign homework, and guide patients through exercises—rather than passive. And they help people across the full spectrum of severity, from those with diagnosed mental disorders to those navigating difficult life transitions or seeking personal growth.

At its core, therapy is a collaborative relationship in which a trained professional helps a person understand and change patterns of thinking, feeling, and behaving that cause distress or impairment. The therapist brings expertise in psychological processes and changing techniques. The patient brings knowledge of their own life, goals, and values. Together, they work toward outcomes the patient has chosen.

Therapy is not advice-giving, though therapists may offer suggestions. It is not friendship, though the relationship shares some qualities with friendship. It is not a place to vent without purpose, though expressing emotion is often part of the work. It is not a way to have someone tell you what to do, though it may help you discover what you truly want.

The therapeutic relationship is unique in several respects. It is entirely focused on the patient's wellbeing, the therapist's needs and problems do not enter the room. It is confidential, allowing disclosure that might be risky in other relationships. It has boundary, existing within clear limits of time and role that provides safety. And it is temporary by design, aiming to help patients develop capacities they will carry forward after therapy ends.

The Evidence Base: What Works?

A question patients reasonably ask is whether therapy actually works. The answer, supported by decades of research involving thousands of studies and hundreds of thousands of patients, is yes— therapy works, and for many conditions it works as well as or better than medication.

Meta-analyses, which combine results from many studies to reach more reliable conclusions, consistently find that psychotherapy produces large effects for depression, anxiety disorders, and many other conditions. Patients who receive therapy improve substantially more than those who receive no treatment or placebo treatments. For some conditions, like panic disorder and specific phobias, therapy is the most effective treatment available. For others, like moderate depression, therapy and medication produce comparable results.

Perhaps more important than the average effect is that therapy works for most people who engage with it. Not everyone improves— some patients do not respond, and a small percentage may even deteriorate—but the majority experience meaningful benefit. This success rate compares favorably with treatments in other areas of medicine.

The effects of therapy also tend to be durable. While medication effects typically persist only as long as medication is continued, the skills and insights gained in therapy often produce lasting change. Studies following patients for years after therapy ends find that benefits are maintained, and that some therapies reduce the risk of future episodes of illness. This durability represents a significant advantage over treatments that must be continued indefinitely.

Not all therapies are equally supported by evidence. Some approaches have been tested extensively and found effective; others have been tested and found ineffective; still others have simply not been studied adequately. Patients seeking therapy should inquire about the evidence supporting the approach their therapist uses, particularly for their specific concerns.

Cognitive Behavioral Therapy: **Changing Thoughts, Changing Lives**

Among the most thoroughly researched and widely practiced forms of therapy is cognitive behavioral therapy, commonly called CBT. Developed in the 1960s and 1970s by Aaron Beck and others, CBT rests on a simple but powerful insight: our thoughts shape our feelings and behaviors, and by changing maladaptive thoughts, we can change how we feel and act.

The cognitive model proposes that psychological distress arises not directly from events but from our interpretations of events. Two people experiencing the same setback may respond very differently depending on how they think about it. One who interprets a job rejection as evidence of permanent inadequacy will feel devastated; another who sees it as a single disappointment in a long career will feel temporarily sad but recover quickly. CBT teaches patients to identify the interpretations driving their distress and to evaluate and modify those interpretations.

A depressed patient might hold the belief that they are worthless and that nothing will ever improve. In CBT, the therapist would help the patient recognize this thought as a hypothesis rather than a fact, examine the evidence for and against it, consider alternative perspectives, and develop more balanced ways of thinking. The patient might discover that their belief in their worthlessness is based on selective attention to failures while ignoring successes, or on holding themselves to impossibly high standards that they would never apply to others.

Beyond thought modification, CBT emphasizes behavioral change. Actions affect emotions just as thoughts do. A depressed patient who has withdrawn from activities and relationships loses opportunities for pleasure and accomplishment, deepening the depression. CBT includes behavioral activation—systematically reengaging with meaningful activities—as a core component. An anxious patient who avoids feared situations never learns that those situations are manageable; CBT includes gradual exposure to feared scenarios, building confidence through experience.

CBT is typically structured and time limited. A course of treatment might involve twelve to twenty sessions over several months, following a progression from assessment through skill-building to application and relapse prevention. Sessions have agendas, homework is assigned between sessions, and progress is monitored systematically. This structure appeals to patients who prefer a practical, goal-oriented approach.

The evidence supporting CBT is extensive. It has been shown effective for depression, generalized anxiety disorder, panic disorder, social anxiety disorder, obsessive-compulsive disorder, post-traumatic stress disorder, eating disorders, insomnia, chronic pain, and many other conditions. For some of these, CBT is the first-line treatment recommended by clinical guidelines. Its effectiveness has been demonstrated across cultures, age groups, and delivery formats.

CBT has also proven adaptable. Specialized versions have been developed for specific conditions—exposure and response prevention for OCD, trauma-focused CBT for PTSD, CBT for insomnia. The core principles remain consistent while techniques are tailored to specific problems.

Beyond CBT: Other Evidence-Based Approaches

While CBT may be the most researched therapy, it is not the only effective approach. Several other therapies have substantial evidence supporting their use, and some may be better suited to particular patients or problems.

Interpersonal therapy, developed originally for depression, focuses on the patient's relationships and social context. It identifies problems in four domains—grief, role transitions, role disputes, and interpersonal deficits—and helps patients address these problems through improved communication and relationship skills. Interpersonal therapy has been shown effective for depression comparable to

CBT and medications and has been adapted for other conditions including eating disorders and anxiety.

Psychodynamic therapy, descended from but distinct from classical psychoanalysis, explores how past experiences, unconscious processes, and relationship patterns contribute to current difficulties. Modern psychodynamic approaches are more focused and time-limited than the caricature of endless analysis, while retaining attention to emotional depth and the therapeutic relationship. Research has demonstrated effectiveness for depression, anxiety, and personality-related difficulties, with some evidence that benefits continue to grow after therapy ends.

Dialectical behavior therapy, originally developed for borderline personality disorder, combines cognitive behavioral techniques with acceptance strategies and mindfulness practices. It teaches skills in four areas: mindfulness, distress tolerance, emotion regulation, and interpersonal effectiveness. Research has demonstrated its effectiveness not only for borderline personality disorder but also for chronic suicidality, self-harm, and emotional dysregulation across diagnostic categories.

Acceptance and commitment therapy emphasizes psychological flexibility— the ability to be present, open to experience, and engaged in value-driven action regardless of difficult thoughts and feelings. Rather than trying to change thoughts, it helps patients change their relationship to thoughts, accepting them as mental events without being controlled by them. Evidence supports its effectiveness for depression, anxiety, chronic pain, and various other conditions.

Eye movement desensitization and reprocessing, or EMDR, is a specialized treatment for trauma in which patients process traumatic memories while engaging in bilateral stimulation, typically by following the therapist's moving finger with their eyes. Despite initial skepticism about its mechanism, research has established EMDR as effective for PTSD, comparable to trauma-focused CBT.

Mindfulness-based therapies incorporate meditation practices into psychological treatment. Mindfulness-based cognitive therapy combines mindfulness training with cognitive therapy principles and has been shown to reduce relapse risk in recurrent depression. Mindfulness-based stress reduction has demonstrated benefits for anxiety, chronic pain, and general wellbeing.

This sampling represents only a portion of approaches with research support. The diversity of effective therapies suggests that multiple paths lead to psychological health, and that matching treatment to patient may be as important as selecting the single "best" therapy.

COMMON FACTORS: What Makes Any Therapy Work

Given the variety of effective therapies, researchers have long asked whether common elements explain their shared effectiveness. The answer appears to be yes—certain factors present across therapies may account for a substantial portion of therapeutic benefit.

The therapeutic alliance— the quality of the relationship between therapist and patient, including agreement on goals, agreement on tasks, and emotional bond—is the most robust predictor of outcome across therapy types. Patients who feel understood, respected, and connected to their therapist improve more than those who do not, regardless of the specific techniques used. This finding underscores that therapy is fundamentally a human relationship, not merely a set of procedures.

Positive expectations also matter. Patients who believe therapy will help them tend to improve more than those who are skeptical. This is not simply placebo effect—the therapy is doing real work—

but hope and expectation mobilize patients' own capacities for change.

Certain therapist qualities predict better outcomes: warmth, empathy, genuineness, and the ability to form strong working relationships. These qualities matter more than the therapist's specific theoretical orientation. A warm therapist practicing one approach may achieve better results than a cold therapist practicing another, even if the second approach has stronger research support on average.

Patient engagement is equally important. Patients who attend sessions consistently, complete homework assignments, and actively participate in the therapeutic process improve more than those who are passive or inconsistent. Therapy requires effort, and patients who invest that effort reap greater rewards.

Finally, the provision of a coherent framework for understanding one's problems and a ritual for addressing them appears beneficial regardless of the specific framework or ritual. Having an explanation for suffering—even if different therapies offer different explanations —and a structured procedure for relief may activate healing processes that transcend particular techniques.

These common factors do not mean that specific techniques are unimportant. For certain conditions, specific techniques appear essential— exposure for anxiety disorders, for instance, or behavioral activation for depression. But the relationship context in which techniques are delivered, and the broader healing elements present across approaches, likely contribute substantially to outcomes.

FINDING the Right Therapist

Given the importance of the therapeutic relationship, finding a therapist with whom one can connect is crucial. This is both a prac-

tical challenge—good therapists are in short supply in many areas—
and a personal one—different patients will connect better with
different therapists.

Training and credentials matter. Therapists may be psychologists,
social workers, counselors, marriage and family therapists, or psychiatrists, among other professional categories. Each profession has its
own training requirements, licensing standards, and scope of practice. Within professions, specialization varies—some therapists focus
on particular conditions, age groups, or treatment approaches.
Patients should seek therapists with training and experience relevant
to their concerns.

Evidence-based practice matters. As noted earlier, not all therapy
approaches have equal evidence supporting them. Patients can ask
potential therapists about their approach and the evidence behind it.
Therapists who cannot articulate an evidence-informed rationale for
their work may not be providing the most effective treatment.

But credentials and approach are not everything. The personal
connection between patient and therapist matters enormously. A first
session is an opportunity to assess whether the therapist seems
understanding, whether their style feels compatible, and whether the
patient can imagine developing trust over time. If the fit does not feel
right, it is reasonable to try a different therapist.

Practical considerations also play a role. Location, scheduling,
cost, and insurance coverage affect which therapists are accessible.
Telehealth options, which expanded dramatically during the
COVID-19 pandemic, have made therapy available to many who
previously faced geographic barriers. Some patients prefer the convenience of video sessions; others value the interpersonal richness of
in-person meetings.

For patients with specific conditions, specialized treatment may
be important. A patient with OCD benefits from a therapist trained in

exposure and response prevention. A patient with PTSD may need a therapist skilled in trauma-focused approaches. A patient with an eating disorder may require treatment from someone experienced with these complex conditions. General therapists, however skilled, may lack the expertise needed for certain problems.

THERAPY in the Digital Age

Technology is transforming how therapy is delivered, extending its reach and creating new possibilities for treatment.

Telehealth therapy—sessions conducted via video rather than in person—has become mainstream. Research conducted during and after the pandemic confirms that telehealth therapy is effective for many conditions, with outcomes comparable to in-person treatment. For patients in rural areas, those with mobility limitations, those with demanding schedules, and those who simply prefer convenience, telehealth removes barriers that previously prevented access to care.

Self-guided digital programs offer another option. Computerized CBT programs lead users through therapeutic content and exercises without a human therapist. Some incorporate interactive elements, personalization based on user responses, and prompts to complete exercises. Research supports their effectiveness for mild to moderate depression and anxiety, though effect sizes are generally smaller than therapist-delivered treatment and dropout rates are higher. They may serve as a first step for those with less severe symptoms or as a supplement to traditional therapy.

Smartphone apps provide continuous access to therapeutic tools. Apps for mindfulness meditation, mood tracking, anxiety management, and various other purposes are widely available. Quality varies enormously—some apps are based on evidence-based approaches and have been evaluated in research; many have not. Patients should seek apps with clear evidence bases, and clinicians increasingly incorporate vetted apps into treatment plans.

Artificial intelligence is beginning to enter the therapeutic space. Chatbots that simulate therapeutic conversations can provide immediate, unlimited access to supportive interaction. Early versions were limited in their capabilities, but advances in AI are producing more sophisticated systems capable of more natural conversation. Whether AI can provide the relational elements that appear central to therapy's effectiveness remains an open question. Current AI tools are best understood as supplements to human treatment rather than replacements for it.

Virtual reality offers possibilities for exposure therapy, allowing patients to confront feared situations in controlled, immersive environments. A patient with fear of flying can experience a virtual airplane takeoff; a patient with social anxiety can practice public speaking before a virtual audience. VR-based exposure has shown effectiveness in research and is beginning to enter clinical practice.

These technologies raise questions about the future of therapy. Will human therapists become less necessary as digital tools improve? Will the relational elements that appear central to therapy be replicated or replaced by technology? Will digital access democratize mental healthcare or create new divides between those who receive human attention and those who receive algorithmic interaction?

Predictions are difficult, but some observations seem warranted. Technology is most likely to extend rather than replace human therapy, reaching patients who would otherwise go untreated and supplementing therapist visits with between-session support. The deepest therapeutic work—addressing trauma, transforming relationship patterns, working through existential struggles—will likely continue to require human presence. But for skill-building, psychoeducation, and support for mild to moderate symptoms, technology may increasingly play a role.

Combining Therapy and Medication

For many conditions, the combination of therapy and medication produces better outcomes than either used alone. Understanding how these modalities complement each other help patients and clinicians make informed treatment decisions.

The mechanisms of therapy and medication differ. Medication alters brain chemistry directly; therapy changes patterns of thought and behavior through learning and experience. Yet both ultimately produce changes in the brain—new connections, altered activity patterns, modified emotional responses. The idea that medication is biological while therapy is merely psychological is outdated; therapy is as biological as medication, working through experience-dependent brain plasticity rather than exogenous chemicals.

For depression, research has compared medication, therapy, and their combination extensively. Either treatment alone helps most patients with mild to moderate depression. For severe depression, combination treatment appears superior to either alone. For preventing relapse, therapy—particularly cognitive therapy—may have advantages over medication alone, as the skills learned persist after treatment ends.

For anxiety disorders, the picture varies by condition. For specific phobias, exposure-based therapy is the treatment of choice; medication adds little. For panic disorder and social anxiety, both therapy and medication are effective; combination may offer modest additional benefit. For OCD, exposure and response prevention therapy is particularly effective and should be part of treatment regardless of whether medication is used.

For PTSD, trauma-focused therapies like prolonged exposure and EMDR are first-line treatments. Medications can reduce symptoms but appear less effective than therapy at producing lasting recovery. Combination treatment is reasonable, particularly for patients with severe symptoms or comorbid conditions.

For conditions like bipolar disorder and schizophrenia, medication is typically essential, but therapy adds significant value. Therapy helps patients understand and adhere to medication regimens, develop coping skills for residual symptoms, rebuild functioning, and process the experience of living with serious mental illness.

As discussed in the previous chapter, the new pharmacology is creating treatments that work synergistically with therapy in new ways. Medications that enhance neuroplasticity may make the brain more responsive to therapeutic learning. Psychedelic-assisted therapy combines a medication experience with intensive psychological processing. The integration of pharmacology and psychology is tighter than ever before.

Patients considering combined treatment should ideally receive coordinated care. When a psychiatrist prescribes medication and a separate therapist provides therapy, the two clinicians should communicate about the treatment plan. When a single provider offers both—as some psychiatrists do—coordination is simpler, but depth of psychological expertise may vary. The optimal arrangement depends on the specific clinicians available, the patient's condition, and practical considerations.

THERAPY Across the Lifespan

Psychotherapy is not one-size-fits-all. Effective treatment looks different for children, adolescents, adults, and older adults, reflecting developmental differences in cognition, social context, and presenting concerns.

Therapy for children typically involves parents substantially. Young children may not be able to articulate their internal experiences or engage in abstract therapeutic conversations. Treatment often works through play, through behavioral interventions that parents implement at home, and through changes to the child's environment. Parent training is a first-line treatment for behavioral problems in young children; the child may not even attend many sessions. As children grow older, they can participate more directly, but parents remain important partners.

Adolescence brings unique challenges. Teenagers are developing identity, navigating complex social worlds, and seeking autonomy from parents— all while their brains undergo dramatic development. Therapy with adolescents must respect their growing independence while recognizing their ongoing need for family support. Conditions like depression, anxiety, eating disorders, and self-harm often emerge during adolescence. Effective therapies address both the adolescent's individual experience and the family dynamics that may contribute to or be affected by the problem.

Adult therapy encompasses the widest range of concerns and approaches. Adults seek therapy for mental health conditions, relationship problems, work difficulties, life transitions, personal growth, and countless other reasons. The diversity of adult experience means that different therapeutic approaches may be appropriate for different patients and problems.

Older adults have long been underserved by psychotherapy, though this is changing. Depression and anxiety are common in later life, often triggered by losses, health problems, and the challenges of aging. Grief, adjustment to retirement, coping with medical illness, and issues around mortality and meaning may bring older adults to therapy. Therapists working with older adults must be knowledge-able about late-life developmental issues and may need to adapt techniques for cognitive or sensory changes.

Throughout the lifespan, therapy must be culturally informed. Patients bring their cultural backgrounds, values, and experiences to treatment. Effective therapists attend to cultural context, recognize how culture shapes the expression and experience of distress, and adapt their approach accordingly. What constitutes effective communication, appropriate emotional expression, and desirable outcomes may vary across cultural groups.

WHEN THERAPY IS NOT WORKING

Not everyone responds to therapy, and when treatment is not producing expected benefits, honest assessment is needed.

The first question is whether the therapy has been given adequate time. Psychological change takes time, and impatience can lead to premature abandonment of potentially effective treatment. Most therapy research suggests that significant improvement typically occurs within eight to twenty sessions for many conditions, though some patients require longer treatment.

The second question is whether the patient is fully engaged. Attending sessions is necessary but not sufficient; patients who complete homework, practice skills outside sessions, and bring genuine effort to the work improve more than those who passively wait for the therapist to fix them. If engagement has been limited, addressing barriers to participation may restart progress.

The third question is whether the therapy approach is appro-priate for the patient's problems. A patient with PTSD receiving supportive counseling without trauma-focused intervention may not improve, not because therapy doesn't work for PTSD but because the

specific therapy being provided is not what works. Seeking a therapist with specialized training may help.

The fourth question is whether the therapeutic relationship is
adequate. If the patient does not feel connected to or understood by
the therapist, changing therapists may be appropriate. The research
on common factors suggests that relationship quality matters
substantially.

The fifth question is whether something else is getting in the way.
Active substance use, ongoing abuse, severe life stressors, or
untreated medical conditions can prevent therapy from working.
Addressing these barriers may be necessary before psychological
treatment can be effective.

Finally, for some patients, therapy alone may be insufficient. The
combination with medication, the use of intensive treatment
programs, or the consideration of novel approaches may be
warranted. Lack of response to one form of treatment does not mean
all treatment will fail.

THE LIMITS of Therapy

Therapy is powerful but not omnipotent. Honest acknowledgment of its limits helps set appropriate expectations.

Therapy cannot change unchangeable circumstances. If distress
arises from poverty, discrimination, chronic illness, or irreversible
loss, therapy cannot eliminate the source of suffering. What it can do
is help patients cope with circumstances, find meaning despite adversity, and identify aspects of their situation that may be changeable.

Therapy cannot transform personality wholesale. While therapy
can help modify maladaptive patterns and reduce personality-related
difficulties, it works with the fundamental temperament the patient
brings. An introverted person will not become an extrovert through

therapy, nor should they expect to. Therapy helps patients work with who they are, not become someone else entirely.

Therapy cannot force change on an unwilling participant. A patient who attends only because a spouse demanded it, or who fundamentally does not believe therapy can help, is unlikely to benefit fully. Motivation and readiness for change are important ingredients in therapeutic success.

Therapy cannot compensate for systemic problems in a patient's life. If someone is struggling primarily because of an abusive relationship, an exploitative job, or a toxic community environment, therapy can support them but cannot substitute for changing or leaving the harmful situation. Sometimes therapeutic work helps patients find the courage to make difficult life changes.

Therapy takes time and effort. Quick fixes for deep-seated problems rarely exist. Patients seeking immediate relief may be disappointed by the gradual nature of therapeutic progress, though the durability of that progress often justifies the investment.

THE THERAPIST'S Perspective

Understanding therapy from the clinician's side may help patients appreciate what happens in the therapeutic relationship.

Therapists undergo extensive training to develop their skills. Doctoral programs in psychology, master's programs in social work and counseling, and psychiatric residencies all include coursework in therapeutic approaches and supervised clinical experience. Beyond initial training, therapists continue to develop through ongoing supervision, continuing education, and their own clinical practice. Expertise accumulates over years.

Therapists use themselves as instruments. Unlike physicians who prescribe medications or surgeons who perform procedures, therapists work primarily through their presence, their listening, their responses, and their ability to create conditions for change. This personal involvement makes the work both rewarding and demanding.

Therapists care about their patients while maintaining professional boundaries. The warmth and concern that effective therapists convey are genuine, not performed. At the same time, the relationship is not friendship; therapists maintain limits that protect both parties and preserve the therapeutic nature of the work.

Therapists experience the work as challenging. Sitting with others' pain, navigating difficult therapeutic moments, tolerating uncertainty about whether treatment is helping, and managing the emotional impact of the work all require effort. Many therapists receive their own therapy or supervision to process the demands of clinical practice.

Therapists vary in quality. Like any profession, some practitioners are more skilled than others. Patients who sense that their therapist is inadequate should trust that perception. Seeking a more competent clinician is appropriate when the current treatment is not working.

INTEGRATION: **A Whole-Person Approach**

The most effective treatment often addresses multiple dimensions of a patient's life simultaneously. The integration of therapy with medication, lifestyle change, social support, and attention to meaning and purpose may produce outcomes superior to any single intervention.

Physical health affects mental health. Sleep problems, lack of exercise, poor nutrition, and chronic medical conditions all influence psychological wellbeing. Therapy that addresses only thoughts and behaviors while ignoring the body misses important contributors to distress. Integrated treatment may include attention to sleep hygiene, encouragement of physical activity, and coordination with medical providers.

Social connection affects mental health. Loneliness and social isolation are risk factors for depression and anxiety; supportive relationships are protective. Therapy often works on relationship skills and may encourage patients to build or repair social connections.

Meaning and purpose affect mental health. Patients who lack a sense that their lives matter, who feel disconnected from values and goals, often struggle regardless of symptom reduction. Some therapeutic approaches address meaning directly; others assume that meaning issues will resolve as symptoms improve. Either way, attention to what makes life worth living is part of comprehensive treatment.

Spiritual or religious resources may support recovery for some patients. For those with faith traditions, spiritual practices and communities can provide comfort, meaning, and support. Therapists need not share patients' beliefs to respect and incorporate these resources into treatment.

The goal of integrated treatment is not merely symptom reduction but human flourishing. Patients deserve not just relief from distress but lives of meaning, connection, and satisfaction. Therapy at its best contributes to this larger vision.

The Future of Psychotherapy

Psychotherapy will continue to evolve in the coming decades. Several trends are likely to shape its future.

Research will continue to refine and develop therapeutic approaches. Better understanding of mechanisms of change will allow treatments to be optimized. New therapies will emerge, and existing therapies will be adapted for new populations and problems.

Technology will play an increasing role. Digital tools will extend the reach of therapy, provide between-session support, and enable new forms of treatment. The balance between human and technological elements will shift, though human presence is likely to remain important for the deepest therapeutic work.

Integration with other treatments will deepen. The combination of therapy with medication, neurostimulation, and novel approaches like psychedelic-assisted treatment will become more sophisticated. The artificial boundary between biological and psychological treatment will fade.

Access will remain a challenge and a priority. The shortage of trained therapists, particularly in underserved areas, will require creative solutions—including technology, task-shifting to less specialized providers, and policy changes to support mental healthcare.

Personalization will advance. Better methods for matching patients to treatments will improve outcomes. Understanding which therapy works best for which patient will move from clinical intuition toward empirical precision.

Through all these changes, the core of therapy will likely remain: one person helping another to understand themselves, to change what can be changed, and to live as fully as possible with what cannot.

CONCLUSION: **The Healing Relationship**

Psychotherapy works because human beings are fundamentally relational creatures, shaped by their connections with others and capable of changing through new relational experiences. The therapeutic relationship offers something rare: focused, nonjudgmental attention from someone trained to help. In that relationship, patterns can be examined, new ways of thinking and behaving can be practiced, and growth that seemed impossible can occur.

Therapy is not magic, and it is not easy. It requires effort from patients and skill from therapists. It takes time—months of weekly sessions for many conditions. It does not work for everyone, and it cannot solve all problems.

But for millions of people, therapy has been the path to recovery from depression, freedom from anxiety, healing from trauma, and transformation of self-defeating patterns. The evidence for its effectiveness is clear; the mechanisms by which it works are increasingly understood; the methods for delivering it are continuously improving.

If you are considering therapy, the research supports giving it a try. If you have tried therapy and not found it helpful, that does not mean therapy cannot help—it may mean you need a different therapist, a different approach, or additional treatment. If you are currently in therapy, your engagement and effort are essential to your progress.

The ancient insight that talking helps is now backed by modern science. The healing relationship, whether called counseling or therapy or simply good conversation, remains one of the most powerful tools we have for reducing suffering and promoting human flourishing.

KEY POINTS **for Patients and Families**

Psychotherapy is a structured form of treatment delivered by trained professionals, distinct from casual conversation or advice-giving.

Research demonstrates that therapy is effective for many conditions, with benefits often comparable to medication and more durable after treatment ends.

Multiple forms of therapy have been shown effective. Cognitive behavioral therapy is among the most researched, but interpersonal therapy, psychodynamic therapy, dialectical behavior therapy, and others also have strong evidence.

Common factors—the therapeutic relationship, positive expectations, patient engagement— contribute to outcomes across therapy types.

Finding a therapist who is both competent and good personal fit is important for successful treatment.

Technology is extending the reach of therapy through telehealth, apps, and digital programs, though human presence remains important for many patients.

Combining therapy with medication often produces better outcomes than alone, especially for severe conditions.

Therapy looks different across the lifespan, with children, adolescents, adults, and older adults each having unique needs.

When therapy is not working, honest assessment of engagement, approach, relationship, and barriers can guide next steps.

The goal of therapy is not just symptom reduction but human flourishing—lives of meaning, connection, and satisfaction.

QUESTIONS for Your Healthcare Provider

1. What type of therapy do you practice, and what is the evidence supporting it for my concerns?
2. How many sessions might I need, and what should I expect the process to look like?
3. How will we know if therapy is working?

4. Should I consider combining therapy with medication?

5. What can I do between sessions to get the most from treatment?

6. How do you approach cultural factors that might be relevant to my treatment?

7. What happens if I don't feel good fit?

8. Are there telehealth options if in-person sessions are difficult?

9. Are there specialized treatments I should consider for my specific condition?

10. What are realistic goals for therapy given my situation?

∼

PART V

Concluding Thoughts

15

WISDOM IN PRESCRIBING
ART WITHIN SCIENCE

Beyond the Algorithm

Throughout this volume, we have explored the science of psychopharmacology— the mechanisms by which medications alter brain chemistry, the evidence supporting their use, the new frontiers being opened by novel treatments. We have examined molecules, receptors, neural circuits, and clinical trials. This scientific foundation is essential. Without it, prescribing becomes guesswork, and patients are subjected to treatments based on fashion or intuition rather than evidence.

But science alone does not make a good prescriber. The physician who knows every mechanism and has memorized every trial result may still fail patients if that knowledge is not applied with wisdom. Wisdom in prescribing means knowing when to start medication and when to wait, when to persist with a treatment and when to change course, how to communicate about medications in ways that promote adherence and realistic expectations, how to balance benefits against risks for this particular patient, and how to integrate pharmacological treatment into a broader vision of healing and flourishing.

This final chapter addresses what cannot be reduced to algorithms or guidelines. It explores the judgment, humility, and humanity that distinguish adequate prescribing from excellent prescribing. For patients, it offers insight into what to seek in a prescriber and how to participate wisely in decisions about medication. For clinicians, it offers reflection on the art that must accompany science. For all readers, it attempts to articulate a philosophy of psychopharmacology that honors both the power and the limits of medication.

The Limits of What We Know

Wisdom begins with epistemic humility—honest acknowledgment of the boundaries of our knowledge.

Psychiatry has made remarkable progress. We have medications that genuinely help millions of people. We understand far more about the brain than we did a generation ago. We have methods for testing treatments rigorously and distinguishing what works from what merely seems to work.

Yet our knowledge remains incomplete. We do not fully understand the pathophysiology of any major psychiatric condition. Our diagnostic categories are descriptive rather than etiological— we group symptoms together without knowing whether they share underlying causes. Our medications were largely discovered by accident, and our understanding of why they work remains partial. We cannot predict with confidence which patient will respond to which medication.

The honest prescriber holds this uncertainty in mind. When explaining a medication to a patient, they convey what is known without overstating certainty. They acknowledge when they are making educated guesses rather than following proven algorithms. They remain open to being wrong.

This humility is not weakness; it is accuracy. The prescriber who speaks with false confidence may temporarily reassure patients but ultimately undermines trust when predictions fail to materialize. The prescriber who acknowledges uncertainty while conveying genuine expertise creates space for the collaborative relationship that medication management requires.

Humility also means recognizing the limits of medication itself. Psychiatric medications are powerful tools, but they are not cures. They manage symptoms rather than eliminating diseases. They work imperfectly, helping some patients dramatically, others modestly, and some not at all. They have side effects that may limit their utility. They are one component of treatment, not the whole of it.

The wise prescriber neither oversells medication as a solution to all problems nor undersells it as mere symptom suppression. They help patients develop realistic expectations—hope grounded in evidence rather than either therapeutic nihilism or magical thinking.

The Whole Person, Not Just the Diagnosis

A prescription is written for a person, not a diagnosis. The same condition in different people may call for different treatments, and the same medication may serve different purposes in different contexts.

Consider depression. One depressed patient is a young professional with a first episode triggered by job loss, good social support, and high motivation for psychotherapy. Another is an elderly widow with recurrent depression, multiple medical comorbidities, limited mobility, and no interest in talking treatment. A third is a new mother experiencing postpartum depression while breastfeeding. A fourth is a teenager whose depression coexists with substance use and self-harm.

All four carry the same diagnosis, but wisdom requires different approaches. The first might reasonably try therapy alone initially, reserving medication for partial response. The second might need medication as a primary intervention, with careful attention to drug interactions and tolerability in an older body. The third requires consideration of infant exposure through breast milk. The fourth needs integrated treatment addressing multiple problems simultaneously.

Beyond diagnosis, the prescriber must understand the patient's life context. What are their responsibilities and constraints? A medication which causes sedation may be unacceptable for someone operating heavy machinery. One, requiring strict dietary restrictions may be impractical for someone with chaotic living circumstances. A treatment demanding frequent monitoring may be inaccessible for someone without transportation.

What are their values and preferences? Some patients strongly prefer to avoid medication if possible; others want medication and find psychotherapy burdensome. Some prioritize rapid relief even if side effects are likely; others prefer gentler approaches even if improvement takes longer. These preferences matter not just ethically but practically; patients who receive treatments aligned with their values are more likely to engage with and benefit from those treatments.

What is the meaning of medication for this patient? For some, taking psychiatric medication represents acceptance of illness and a step toward recovery. For others, it feels like failure, weakness, or loss of self. These meanings, often unspoken, profoundly influence adherence with and response to medications. The wise prescriber explores meaning rather than assuming it.

What resources do the patient have for treatment? Social support, financial stability, access to therapy, and general coping capacity all influence how medication fits into the treatment picture. A medication that works well when combined with therapy and lifestyle changes may be insufficient alone.

THE ART of Starting

Initiating medication is a decision that warrants careful consideration. The wise prescriber neither rushes to prescribe at the first sign of distress nor withholds medication when it is clearly indicated.

Timing matters. For mild to moderate symptoms, particularly in first episodes, a period of watchful waiting or initial trial of non-pharmacological treatment may be appropriate. Many patients improve with therapy, lifestyle changes, time, or resolution of precipitating stressors. Starting medication immediately may subject patients to side effects and risks that were not necessary.

Yet delay has costs too. Patients suffering from severe symptoms deserve prompt relief. Untreated illness can worsen, become entrenched, or lead to cascading consequences in relationships, work, and health. The prescriber must weigh the risks of premature treatment against the risks of inadequate treatment.

When medication is indicated, the choice of agent requires thought. First-line medications are called first-line because they have the best balance of efficacy, tolerability, and safety for most patients. But "most patients" does not mean every patient. Individual history, family history of medication response, comorbid conditions, concomitant medications, and specific symptom profiles may all influence the optimal choice.

Starting doses and titration schedules also require judgment. The maxim "start low, go slow" protects against early side effects that might lead patients to abandon treatment. But excessively slow titration may delay benefit and lose patients to discouragement. The right pace depends on symptom severity, patient sensitivity, and practical constraints.

Clear communication at the start sets the stage for successful treatment. Patients need to understand what the medication is expected to do, how long it may take to work, what side effects might occur, what to do if problems arise, and what the plan is if this medication does not help. They need to know that finding the right treatment sometimes requires trial and adjustment. They need permission to call with questions and concerns.

The prescriber who takes time for this conversation invests in adherence. The prescriber who hands over a prescription with minimal explanation should not be surprised when patients take medication erratically, stop at the first side effect, or never fill the prescription at all.

The Art of Waiting

After starting medication, a period of uncertainty follows. Most psychiatric medications do not work immediately. Antidepressants typically require weeks before full effect; mood stabilizers may need months to demonstrate their value in preventing episodes; even faster-acting medications take time to optimize.

This waiting period is challenging for everyone. Patients continue to suffer while wondering whether the medication is helping. Prescribers cannot know whether early non-response predicts ultimate failure or simply reflects the normal timeline of treatment. The temptation to change medications prematurely is strong.

Wisdom requires patience without passivity. The prescriber who abandons medication after two weeks has not given it a fair trial. But the prescriber who rigidly insists on twelve weeks before any modification ignores useful information and prolongs unnecessary suffering.

Monitoring during this period serves multiple purposes. It allows early detection of side effects or worsening. It provides support and hope during a difficult time. It builds the relationship that will be needed for long-term management. And it generates information that guides next steps.

The question of what constitutes adequate response is not always clear-cut. Some improvement is better than none, but partial response leaves open the question of whether to optimize the current medication, add another, or switch entirely. The patient's perspective on what is acceptable matters here—some patients are satisfied with partial relief while others expect complete remission.

The Art of Adjusting

When initial treatment is inadequate, adjustment is needed. The wise prescriber approaches this process systematically while remaining flexible.

The first question is whether the medication has been given a fair trial. Has the dose been optimized? Has sufficient time elapsed? Has the patient actually taken the medication as prescribed? These questions must be answered before concluding that the medication has failed.

If the trial has been adequate and response is insufficient, several options exist: increasing the dose if room remains within the therapeutic range, adding a second medication to augment the first, switching to a different medication, or adding non-pharmacological treatment. Each option has advantages and disadvantages. The choice depends on how much the current medication has helped, the nature of residual symptoms, the patient's tolerance of current side effects, and preferences about polypharmacy versus switching.

Switching medications means abandoning any benefit the current medication provided and risking that the new medication will be worse. Augmenting preserves current benefit but adds complexity, cost, and potential for drug interactions. There is no universally correct choice; the decision must be individualized.

When switching, the prescriber must manage the transition. Some switches require gradual cross-tapering; others can be done more abruptly. Discontinuation symptoms, drug interactions during the transition, and the potential for relapse during the gap between effective treatments must all be considered.

Throughout this process, documentation matters. Recording what was tried, at what doses, for how long, and with what results creates a treatment history that will be invaluable if the current prescriber changes or if future episodes require new decisions. The patient who can say "I tried medications X, Y, and Z at adequate doses without benefit" is far ahead of one who can only say "I tried a bunch of stuff that didn't work."

THE ART of Continuing

For many patients, long-term or even lifelong medication is appropriate. Conditions like bipolar disorder, recurrent major depression, and schizophrenia typically require maintenance treatment to prevent relapse. Stopping medication often causes the illness to return, sometimes more severely.

Yet long-term treatment brings its own challenges. Side effects that seemed tolerable for a few months may become intolerable over years. The meaning of chronic medication—what it implies about identity, about the permanence of illness—may evolve. Life circumstances change, altering the risk-benefit calculation.

The wise prescriber revisits the treatment plan periodically rather than simply renewing prescriptions indefinitely. Is the medication still necessary? Are there side effects that have been tolerated but not discussed? Has the patient's perspective on treatment changed? Are there new options that were not available when treatment started?

At the same time, the prescriber must help patients resist the temptation to stop medication prematurely. Patients often feel better on medication and conclude they no longer need it, not recognizing that feeling better is the medication's effect. The prescriber must educate about the importance of maintenance treatment for conditions where it is indicated, while respecting autonomy if patients choose differently.

Long-term management also requires attention to general health. Psychiatric medications can affect weight, metabolic function, cardiac health, and other aspects of physical wellbeing. Regular monitoring and proactive management of these effects are part of responsible prescribing.

The Art of Stopping

There comes a time, for some patients, when stopping medication is appropriate. Perhaps it was prescribed for a single episode that has fully remitted. Perhaps side effects have become unacceptable. Perhaps the patient has decided, after full consideration, that they prefer to manage without medication. Perhaps a medication trial has clearly failed.

Stopping requires the same care as starting. Many psychiatric medications cause discontinuation symptoms if stopped abruptly—

antidepressants can produce flu-like symptoms, sensory disturbances, and emotional lability; benzodiazepines can cause dangerous
withdrawal. Gradual tapering is usually necessary.

The prescriber must also prepare the patient for what might
follow. If the medication was suppressing symptoms of an ongoing
illness, those symptoms may return. The patient needs to know the
warning signs of relapse and have a plan for what to do if they occur.
Sometimes a trial of stopping is reasonable, with the understanding
that medication can be restarted if needed.

When medication is stopped because it was not helping, the
prescriber should revisit the diagnosis and treatment plan. Was the
diagnosis correct? Was an adequate trial given? Are there other treatments—pharmacological or otherwise—that should be considered?

COMMUNICATION AS CORE Skill

Throughout all phases of prescribing, communication is central.
The wise prescriber is not merely a technician selecting medications
but a communicator helping patients understand and participate in
their treatment.

Explaining medications in accessible terms requires translating
complex pharmacology into language patients can use. This does not
mean dumbing down or being condescending; it means finding
metaphors and explanations that convey essential information
without unnecessary jargon.

Informed consent is both ethical requirement and therapeutic
tool. Patients who understand what they are taking, why they are
taking it, and what to expect are better partners in treatment. They
recognize expected side effects rather than panicking. They understand why adherence matters. They can participate meaningfully in
decisions about adjustments.

Addressing concerns and misconceptions is part of every prescriber's job. Patients come with fears—of addiction, of personality change, of being "zombified," of long-term harm. Some fears are based on misinformation and can be corrected. Others reflect genuine uncertainties that deserve honest acknowledgment. Still others may be displaced concerns about the illness itself or the meaning of needing treatment.

The prescriber who dismisses patient concerns alienates patients and undermines adherence. The prescriber who addresses concerns with respect and accurate information builds the partnership that effective treatment requires.

Cultural humility matters here too. Attitudes toward medication, mental illness, and medical authority vary across cultures. What constitutes appropriate decision-making—individual autonomy versus family involvement, for instance—differs across communities. The wise prescriber learns about the patient's cultural context and adapts communication accordingly.

When Things Go Wrong

Despite best efforts, things sometimes go wrong. Medications cause unexpected severe side effects. Patients deteriorate despite treatment. Errors occur.

How prescribers respond to adverse events reveal their character. The temptation to become defensive, to blame the patient, or to minimize what happened is understandable but harmful. The wise prescriber acknowledges what has occurred, expresses appropriate concern, works to address the problem, and learns from the experience.

Medication errors—wrong drug, wrong dose, dangerous interactions—happen even to careful prescribers. Systems should be designed to prevent them, but when they occur, transparency is both ethically required and practically wise. Patients who feel their prescriber is honest about mistakes are more forgiving than those who sense concealment.

When a patient fails to respond to treatment after treatment, the prescriber must resist demoralization. Treatment-resistant illness is genuinely difficult; some patients improve only after many trials or not at all. The prescriber's job is to keep trying, to explore options, to maintain hope without making false promises, and to support patients through what may be a long and discouraging process.

Sometimes the wise response is to recognize the limits of one's own expertise and refer to a specialist. Complex cases may benefit from expert consultation. Prescribers who never seek second opinions are overconfident; those who seek them appropriately are practicing good medicine.

Avoiding Common Traps

Experience teaches that certain pitfalls recur. Naming them may help prescribers avoid them.

The trap of treating numbers rather than people leads to adjusting medications based on rating scale scores without attending to the patient's actual experience. Scales are useful tools but not the goal of treatment.

The trap of polypharmacy accumulates medications without clear rationale, adding agents for each symptom without periodically reassessing whether each drug is still contributing. Patients on six or eight medications deserve careful review of whether each addition was justified and remains necessary.

The trap of therapeutic inertia continues unsuccessful treatment too long, out of habit or lack of attention. Patients stable in their suffering receive refill after refill without anyone asking whether they might do better.

The trap of chasing side effects adds medications to treat the side effects of other medications, building a tower of interventions that may ultimately cause more harm than the original symptom warranted.

The trap of false precision adjusts doses by small increments that are unlikely to produce meaningful differences, creating an illusion of fine-tuning where none is possible.

The trap of ignoring context prescribes medications for problems that are fundamentally situational—the patient who is anxious because their job is abusive, depressed because their marriage is failing, or sleepless because they consume caffeine until midnight. Medication cannot substitute for addressing the actual problem.

The trap of countertransference lets the prescriber's feelings about the patient—frustration with "difficult" patients, excessive identification with some patients, discomfort with certain presentations— drive treatment decisions that should be based on clinical judgment.

WISDOM BEYOND MEDICATION

The wisest prescribers recognize that medication is embedded in a larger context of treatment and of life.

Medication works best when combined with psychotherapy for many conditions. The prescriber who ignores therapy deprives patients of benefit. Even when prescribing is the primary role, facilitating access to therapy and supporting engagement with it is part of the job.

Lifestyle factors profoundly affect mental health. Sleep, exercise, nutrition, substance use, social connection, and stress all influence illness course and medication response. The prescriber who addresses only medication while ignoring modifiable lifestyle factors practices incomplete medicine.

Social determinants of health—poverty, discrimination, housing instability, trauma—underlie much psychiatric suffering. Medication cannot fix these problems, but the prescriber should at least recognize them and connect patients with resources that address them.

Meaning, purpose, and hope matter in ways that no medication directly provides. The patient who has reasons to get better, who can envision a future worth living, who feels connected to something larger than their illness, has resources beyond any prescription. The wise prescriber attends to these dimensions of the patient's life.

THE PRESCRIBER-PATIENT RELATIONSHIP

At the heart of wise prescribing is the relationship between prescriber and patient. This relationship is not merely a context in which medication is delivered; it is itself therapeutic.

Patients who trust their prescriber are more likely to take medication as prescribed, report problems honestly, and tolerate the difficulties of treatment. The prescriber's genuine concern, expressed through attention and care over time, contributes to outcomes in ways that cannot be measured by any scale.

This relationship requires investment. Brief medication checks, however necessary in some practice settings, do not build the alliance that supports patients through long-term treatment. Prescribers in high-volume settings must find ways to convey care even in limited time. Those with more time should use it to know their patients as people, not just as bearers of diagnoses.

Continuity matters. The prescriber who follows a patient over years accumulates knowledge of that patient's history, responses, preferences, and life context that cannot be quickly conveyed to a new provider. Systems that fragment care—patients seeing whoever is available, records that do not communicate across settings—undermine the relationships that make prescribing most effective.

Boundaries matter too. The prescriber-patient relationship is professional, not personal. The prescriber's job is to serve the patient's health, not to become the patient's friend, savior, or target of excessive dependency. Maintaining appropriate limits protects both parties and preserves the therapeutic nature of the relationship.

TEACHING the Next Generation

Wisdom cannot be taught directly, but it can be modeled and encouraged.

Trainees learn prescribing partly from textbooks and lectures but mostly from watching their supervisors. The supervisor who demonstrates humility, careful thinking, respectful communication, and genuine concern teaches these qualities more effectively than any curriculum.

Case-based teaching that explores not just what was done but why—including alternatives considered and rejected—develops the reasoning that underlies wise prescribing. The teaching that presents algorithm-following as sufficient produces technicians, not wise clinicians.

Encouraging reflection is essential. The trainee who can articulate what went well and what might have been done differently is developing self-awareness that sustains growth throughout a career. The training program that makes no space for reflection produces prescribers who stop developing when training ends.

Modeling uncertainty is perhaps most important. Supervisors who present themselves as knowing everything convey a false picture of clinical reality and leave trainees unprepared for the ambiguity they will encounter. Supervisors who demonstrate how to think through uncertainty make reasonable decisions despite incomplete information and remain open to being wrong prepare trainees for actual practice.

THE LARGER VISION

Psychopharmacology at its best serves a larger vision: the reduction of suffering and the promotion of flourishing.

Medications relieve symptoms, but relief of symptoms is not the ultimate goal. The goal is to have a life worth living— lives of meaning, connection, creativity, and joy. Sometimes medication is necessary to make such lives possible; sometimes it contributes modestly; sometimes it is irrelevant or even counterproductive.

The wise prescriber holds this larger vision in mind. The question is not only "Is the depression rating scale score improving?" but "Is this person moving toward a life that is good for them?" Sometimes these questions have the same answer; sometimes they diverge.

This vision requires attention to what patients themselves want. Prescribers can offer expertise about medications and their effects, but patients are the experts on their own values and goals. The treatment that optimizes prescriber-defined outcomes may not be the treatment the patient most wants. Shared decision-making, in which clinical expertise and patient values together determine the treatment plan, operationalizes this respect.

CONCLUSION: The Wise Prescriber

What, then, characterizes the wise prescriber?

The wise prescriber knows the science—mechanisms, evidence,

guidelines—but holds this knowledge with appropriate humility, recognizing what remains unknown.

The wise prescriber sees the whole person, not just the diagnosis, and they tailor treatment to the individual's context, values, and preferences.

The wise prescriber communicates clearly, honestly, and respectfully, treating patients as partners rather than passive recipients of treatment.

The wise prescriber exercises patience without passivity, knowing when to wait and when to act, when to persist and when to change course.

The wise prescriber attends to the therapeutic relationship, recognizing that how medication is prescribed matters as much as what is prescribed.

The wise prescriber avoids common traps—polypharmacy without rationale, therapeutic inertia, treating numbers rather than people, ignoring context.

The wise prescriber integrates medication with other treatments and with attention to lifestyle, social context, and meaning.

The wise prescriber keeps learning, recognizing that knowledge evolves and that every patient teaches something new.

The wise prescriber remains connected to the larger purpose of the work: not merely managing illness but supporting patients in building lives worth living.

PSYCHOPHARMACOLOGY IS POWERFUL. The medications discussed throughout this volume have transformed lives, reduced suffering, and made possible recoveries that seemed unimaginable a century ago. The advances on the horizon—personalized medicine, novel mechanisms, treatments that work where current options fail—promise further progress.

But medication is not magic. It works best when prescribed wisely by clinicians who combine scientific knowledge with human understanding, who see patients as people rather than problems, who communicate with honesty and respect, and who recognize that pharmacology is one tool among many in the service of human flourishing.

This volume has offered science. This final chapter has attempted to articulate wisdom. The integration of both—in training, in practice, in the ongoing development of every prescriber—is what patients deserve and what excellent psychiatry requires.

KEY POINTS for Patients and Families

Choose a prescriber who takes time to understand you as a person, not just your diagnosis.

Ask questions about any medication you are prescribed—what it does, what to expect, what the alternatives are. A good prescriber welcomes these questions.

Be honest with your prescriber about how you are taking medication, any side-effects you may be experiencing, and how you feel about treatment. They cannot help you if they do not know what is happening.

Give medications a fair trial before concluding they do not work; but speak up if you are having problems or not improving.

Remember that medication is usually one part of treatment, not the whole of it. Therapy, lifestyle changes, and social support also matter.

If you are not comfortable with your prescriber or feel unheard, seeking a different provider is reasonable. The relationship matters.

Keep a record of what medications you have tried and how they worked. This information is valuable for future treatment decisions.

Understand that finding the right medication sometimes takes time and multiple trials. Persistence usually pays off.

QUESTIONS **for Your Healthcare Provider**

1. What is your approach to prescribing medications—how do you decide what to try and when?
2. How do you think about combining medication with therapy and other treatments?
3. How will we communicate between appointments if I have questions or problems?
4. How do you handle it when patients have concerns about taking medication?
5. What is your approach when a medication is not working well?
6. How do you decide when to stop medication?
7. How do you stay current with new developments in psychopharmacology?
8. What role do my own values and preferences play in treatment decisions?
9. How do you think about the long-term effects of medication?
10. What is your overall philosophy of medication treatment in psychiatry?

～

16

CONCLUSION
WHEN TRUTH BECOMES SPEAKABLE

I n the course of my work, I have come to understand that one of the greatest obstacles to healing is not the intensity of a person's suffering, but the inability—or the fear—to speak about it plainly. People rarely enter the room speaking fluently, in the language of their own distress. They reach for the terms our culture has handed them: depression, anxiety, stress, or the vague, self-protective "I'm fine." These words soften what hurts. They protect what feels fragile. They hide what feels unsayable.

Over the years, I have learned to gently interrupt this familiar pattern. I ask my patients: "Tell me how you suffer but do so without using catchwords. Tell me what it feels like in your body, in your days, in your thoughts."

This request is deceptively simple, but it transforms the encounter. It invites truth where habit once stood.

I explain to them that this difficulty is universal. Almost no one arrives with clear emotional vocabulary. Most people carry shame about their inner life, and shame constricts speech. But when we acknowledge this openly—when we move from the isolated *I* to the shared *we*— shame softens. Suffering becomes less private, less punishing, less defining.

THE SAME PATTERN emerges when I ask about family history. The most common answers are tentative: "not really," "I don't think so," or a quick change of subject. For years, I misinterpreted this as minimization. Now I understand it as a form of protection—a guarding of the family, guarding the self, a fear of what acknowledgment might unleash.

When I gently tell patients that defensiveness is common, that emotional pain becomes more comprehensible—not less—when we widen the lens from individual to family to society, something shifts. A small permission opens. Stories begin to emerge.

THIS PROCESS— this gradual unveiling— has become, for me, a form of applied philosophy. Psychiatry at its best is not merely diagnostic. It is an excavation of meaning.

Nietzsche has been a quiet companion in this understanding. He wrote that honesty— especially honesty about one's suffering— is an act of courage, a confrontation with truths the self often avoids. When I encourage patients to replace labels with lived experience, I am asking them to step outside what Nietzsche called the herd vocabulary—those shared, flattened words that cover complexity with familiarity.

I want them to reclaim their experience in their own language.

The clinical interview becomes, in this way, a small training ground for transformation. Nietzsche wrote of the need to "give style" to one's character—to shape the chaos within into something coherent and true. This is precisely what happens when a patient begins to articulate their pain without apology. They move from being a passive recipient of suffering to an active interpreter of it. Their story becomes theirs again.

THE DEEPER WISDOM I have learned is this: before healing can occur, language must be liberated.

When a person can describe their inner world honestly—without shame, without borrowed labels, without fear of being misunderstood— something powerful happens. Suffering does not vanish, but it becomes more intelligible. It becomes organized, nameable, shareable. And what is shareable becomes survivable.

As conversations unfold in this way, more truth emerges than any checklist could ever uncover. Not because I ask more questions, but because the patient becomes less afraid of their own answers. Empathy becomes the catalyst for revelation. The recognition of shared humanity becomes the antidote to shame.

IF THERE IS ONE TEACHING, I hope the reader carries from this book, it is this: psychiatry is not only a science; it is a dialogue of courage.

Our task is not merely to diagnose disorders, but to cultivate the conditions in which a person can speak truthfully about their life. To help them move from minimization to expression, from isolation to universality, from inherited silence to genealogical understanding.

This is the essence of wisdom in psychiatry.

And in the end, wisdom is not found in labels or protocols, but in the freedom that arises when a person speaks in their own voice and discovers—perhaps for the first time—that their suffering can be met with honesty, dignity, and meaning.

It is in that moment, when truth becomes speakable, that healing truly begins.

ABOUT THE AUTHOR

The author is a psychiatrist and writer, board-certified in adult, child, and adolescent psychiatry, with decades of experience listening to how people describe their suffering. His work explores where psychiatric labels fall short—and how language, shame, and moral assumptions shape inner life.

Drawing on both clinical practice and philosophy, especially Nietzsche, he writes about the psychology of meaning, self-understanding, and human development. He approaches mental health not as a set of formulas, but as a way of learning to see more clearly—without reducing what is seen.

∼

INDEX

www.ingramcontent.com/pod-product-compliance
Lightning Source LLC
Chambersburg PA
CBHW052118270326
41930CB00012B/2673